Reiki Manual

Level Two

Rajesh Nanoo

For orders and enquires, contact
www.rajeshnanoo.com
mrknowable@gmail.com

Of thy dear form,
O Prana,
Of thy very dear form,
Of the healing power
That is thine,
Give unto us,
That we may live!

Atharva Veda

Dr. Rajesh Nanoo MD(AM) had a spiritual inclination from my early days towards occult sciences and music. At first he nurtured his skills in Multimedia and started creating logos, posters and storyboard for various clients. Shortly his attention shifted to the potentials of Reiki and embraced this astonishing healing power. With enthusiasm, he pursued this magnificent profession along with Yoga Therapy and learned other holistic techniques which enabled him to hasten the healing process.

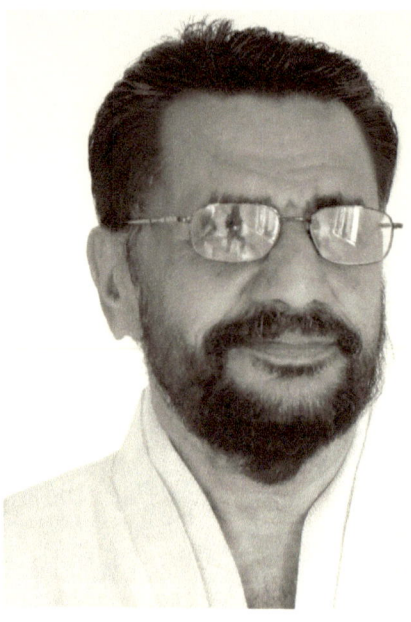

The research done on various philosophies enabled him to come up with training modules on enhancing life skills. He was involved in training people on the secret of working smartly, giving energy healing and teaching relaxation techniques to withstand the stress of the modern society.

Holistic training/healing methodology is a self-help tool to pull us out from difficulties; it has an integral part to play in character making. Rajesh Nanoo have comprehended this truth and crave to extend this awareness for the needy ones for cure and also to renovate their character, thereby let the world recognize the new era of healing/training that has begun by transcending a man completely.

CONTENTS

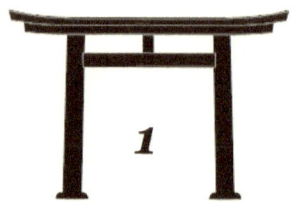

1   *Classification -1*

Human anatomy according to medical science*

The body is made up of many parts all of which work together for the common good of the entire body. There are many different types of cells in the human body. None of these cells function alone, they are part of the larger organism that is called - you (human body).There are many systems in the body. The composition of a system in the body will determine what functions it performs in the body. Systems in a way are specialized parts of our body. There is however co-ordination of the functions of systems of the body. The Human Body has five main senses; Sight, Smell, Taste, Hearing and Touch. Each of these senses detects a feature of the environment and produces nerve signals to carry this information to the brain.

Dozens of different kinds of cells are organized into specialized groups called tissues. Different tissue types are assembled into organs. An organ is a structure that contains at least two different types of tissue functioning together for a common purpose. It is a distinct set of cells within a multi cellular organism that perform a distinct function. Organs include the heart, lungs, brain, eye, stomach, spleen, pancreas, kidneys, liver, intestines, uterus, bladder etc. The skin is the largest organ of the human body. The liver is the largest internal organ of the human body. All organs are made of tissues. Every organ has its own special function. The function of the heart is to keep blood flowing round the body by pumping blood into the blood vessel. Organs, in turn, are organized into systems such as the circulatory, digestive, or nervous systems. All together, these assembled organ systems form the human body. The major systems of the human body are:

1. Cardiovascular system: the blood circulation with heart, arteries and veins
2. Digestive system: processing food with mouth, esophagus, stomach and intestines.
3. Endocrine system: communicating within the body using hormones
4. Excretory system: eliminating wastes from the body
5. Immune system: defending against disease-causing agents
6. Integumentary system: skin, hair and nails
7. Muscular system: moving the body with muscles
8. Nervous system: collecting, transferring and processing information with brain and nerves
9. Reproductive system: the sex organs
10. Respiratory system: the organs used for breathing, the lungs
11. Skeletal system: structural support and protection through bones.
12.

Each system represents different set of organs, they are:

Skeletal	Bones, cartilage, tendons and ligaments.
Cardiovascular(Circulatory)	Heart, blood vessels, erythroblasts
Digestive	Esophagus, stomach, intestines, liver, pancreas
Endocrine	Pituitary, adrenal, thyroid, other ductless glands
Immune	Spleen, thymus, skin, white blood cells

Nervous	Brain regions, peripheral nervous tissue
Reproductive	Testes, ovaries, associated reproductive structures
Respiratory	Lungs, trachea, other air passages
Muscular	Skeletal muscle, cardiac muscle, smooth muscle
Excretory	Kidneys, ureters, bladder and urethra.

1. Skeletal system.

The main role of the skeletal system is to provide support for the body, to protect delicate internal organs and to provide attachment sites for the organs. The Skeleton is the name given to the collection of bones that holds the rest of our body up. When you were born, your skeleton had around 350 bones. By the time you become an adult, you will only have around 206 bones. This is because, as you grow, some of the bones join together to form one bone. Our bones don't simply work on their own will. The bones join together to form joints. Our skeleton is very important to us. It does three major jobs.

1. It protects our vital organs such as the brain, the heart and the lungs.
2. It gives us the shape that we have. Without our skeleton, we would just be a blob of bloodt and tissue on the floor.
3. It allows us to move. Because our muscles are attached to our bones, when our muscles move, they move the bones, and we move.

2. Muscular system

The main role of the muscular system is to provide movement that allows them to move internally and externally. Muscles work in pairs to move limbs and provide the organism with mobility. Muscles also control the movement of materials through some organs, such as the stomach and intestine, and the heart and circulatory system. Muscles are made up of thousands of thin, long, cylindrical cells called muscle fibers. The muscle fibers' highly specialized structure enables the muscles to relax and contract to produce movement. Muscles vary greatly in their shape and size, depending on their function. There are two main types.

1.   Voluntary muscles-under our control and
2.   Involuntary muscles-outside our minds control.

The most astonishing muscle of all is the heart muscle which works incessantly form birth to death.

3. Circulatory system

The main role of the circulatory system is to transport nutrients, gases (such as oxygen and CO_2), hormones and wastes through the body. It consists of heart and blood vessels. Together, these provide a continuous flow of blood to your body, supplying the tissues with oxygen and nutrients. Arteries carry blood away from the heart; veins return blood to the heart. Oxygenated blood is pumped out of the heart through the body's main artery — the aorta. Arteries that branch off the aorta transport blood throughout the body, supplying tissues with oxygen and nutrients. Tiny vessels called capillaries in organs and tissues of the body deliver deoxygenated blood into small veins called venules, which join to form veins. Blood flows through the veins to the body's two main veins (called the vena cavae), which deliver the blood back into the heart.

4. Nervous system

The Nervous System is the most complex and delicate of all the body systems. At the center of the nervous system is the brain. The brain sends and receives messages through a network of nerves. This network of nerves allows the brain to communicate with every part of the body. Nerves transmit information as electrical impulses from one area of the body to another. Some nerves carry information to the brain. This allows us to see, hear, smell, taste and touch. Other nerves carry information from the brain to the muscles to control our body's movement and behavior. It along with the endocrine system, controls physiological processes such as digestion, circulation, etc. Many drugs, such as alcohol and cigarettes, affect the way that our nerves work.

5. Respiratory system

The system is the biological system of any organism that engages in gaseous exchange. Even trees have respiratory systems, taking in carbon dioxide and emitting oxygen. The main role of the respiratory system is to provide gas exchange between the blood and the environment. Primarily, oxygen is absorbed from the atmosphere into the body and carbon dioxide is expelled from the body. The system provides the energy needed by cells of the body. Oxygen in the blood is delivered to body cells, where the oxygen and glucose in the cells undergo a series of reactions to provide energy to cells, and the waste product of this process is carried out of the lungs as carbon dioxide.

6. Digestive system

The main role of the digestive system is to breakdown and absorbs nutrients that are necessary for growth and maintenance. It consists of organs that break down food into components that your body uses for energy and for building and repairing cells and tissues. Food provides us with fuel to live, energy to work and play, and the raw materials to build new cells. All the different varieties of food we eat are broken down by our digestive system and transported to every part of our body by our circulatory system. The main part of the digestive system is the digestive tract. This is like a long tube, some nine meters in total, through the middle of the body. It starts at the mouth, where food and drink enter the body, and finishes at the anus, where leftover food and wastes leave the body.

Food passes down the throat, down through a muscular tube called the esophagus, and into the stomach, where food continues to be broken down. The partially digested food passes into a short tube called the duodenum (first part of the small intestine). The jejunum and ileum are also part of the small intestine. The liver, the gallbladder, and the pancreas produce enzymes and substances that help with digestion in the small intestine. The last section of the digestive tract is the large intestine, which includes the cecum, colon, and rectum. The appendix is a branch off the large intestine; it has no known function. Indigestible remains of food are expelled through the anus.

7. Excretory system

The excretory system is the system of an organism's body that performs the function of excretion. The main role is to filter out cellular wastes, toxins and excess water or nutrients from the circulatory system. The urinary tract is the body system involved in the formation and excretion of urine. The kidneys filter out waste products from the blood. These waste products in combination with water are urine. The urine passes out of the kidneys through two narrow, muscular tubes called ureters. The ureters empty the urine into the bladder, and the urine is then excreted from the body through a tube like structure called the urethra.

8. Endocrine system

The main role of the endocrine system is to relay chemical messages through the body. In conjunction with the nervous system, these chemical messages help control physiological processes such as nutrient absorption, growth, etc. the system is a collection of ductless endocrine glands that produce hormones that regulate the body's growth, metabolism, and sexual development and function. The hormones are released into the bloodstream and transported to tissues and organs throughout your body. It does not include exocrine glands such as salivary glands, sweat glands and glands within the gastrointestinal tract.

The major glands that make up the human endocrine system are the hypothalamus, pituitary, thyroid, parathyroid, adrenals, pineal body, and the reproductive glands - the ovaries and testes. The pancreas is also part of this hormone-secreting system, even though it is also associated with the digestive system because the exocrine part of the pancreas also produces and secretes digestive enzymes into the intestine. Although the endocrine glands are the body's main hormone producers, some non endocrine organs - such as the brain, heart, lungs, kidneys, liver, thymus, skin, and placenta - also produce and release hormones. Glands are:

1. Adrenal glands Divided into 2 regions; secrete hormones that influence the body's metabolism, blood chemicals, and body characteristics, as well as influence the part of the nervous system that is involved in the response and defense against stress.
2. Hypothalamus Activates and controls the part of the nervous system that controls involuntary body functions, the hormonal system, and many body functions, such as regulating sleep and stimulating appetite.
3. Ovaries and testicles Secrete hormones that influence female and male characteristics, respectively.
4. Pancreas Secretes a hormone (insulin) that controls the use

of glucose by the body.
5. Parathyroid glands Secrete a hormone that maintains the calcium level in the blood.
6. Pineal body Involved with daily biological cycles.
7. Pituitary gland Produces a number of different hormones that influence various other endocrine glands.
8. Thymus gland Plays a role in the body's immune system.
9. Thyroid gland Produces hormones that stimulate body heat production, bone growth, and the body's metabolism.

9. Reproductive system

Many parts of human sexual anatomy are homologous between the sexes. The sexual organs of the male are partly visible and partly hidden within the body. The female sexual organs are almost entirely hidden. The main role of the reproductive system is to manufacture cells that allow reproduction. In the male, sperm are created to inseminate egg cells produced in the female.

Reproduction is accomplished by the union of male sperm and the female ovum. In coitus, the male organ ejaculates more than 250 million sperm into the vagina, from which some make their way to the uterus. Ovulation, the release of an egg into the uterus, occurs approximately every 28 days; during the same period the uterus is prepared for the implantation of a fertilized ovum by the action of estrogens. If a male cell fails to unite with a female cell, other hormones cause the uterine wall to slough off during menstruation. From puberty to menopause, the process of ovulation, and preparation, and menstruation is repeated monthly except for periods of pregnancy. The duration of pregnancy is about 280 days. After childbirth, prolactin, a hormone secreted by the pituitary, activates the production of milk.

10. Immune system

The main role of the immune system is to destroy and remove invading microbes and viruses from the body. The body defends itself against foreign proteins and infectious microorganisms by means of a complex dual system that depends on recognizing a portion of the surface pattern of the invader. The two parts of the system are termed cellular immunity, in which lymphocytes are the effective agent, and humoral immunity, based on the action of antibody molecules. Together, all these parts form the body's immune defense system.

11. Integumentary system

The Integumentary system in the human body is comprised of the skin, hair and nails. Its main role is to protect us from heat and cold. The skin is made up of a thin outer layer (called the epidermis) and a thicker inner layer (called the dermis). Below the dermis is the subcutaneous tissue, which contains fat. Buried in the skin are nerves that sense cold, heat, pain, pressure, and touch. Deep within the skin are your sweat glands, which produce perspiration when you are too hot. Hair is a characteristic of all mammals, though in some species hair is absent at certain stages of life. Hair serves a number of different functions. It provides insulation from cold weather and, in some species, from particularly hot weather.

Note – Taken from various Internet sources

Human Anatomy in short

The human body consists of cells, tissues, organs, systems. Cells and tissues make up organs. A system is the combination of organs. There are nine systems in the body. Human body is the combination of all these systems.

Cells make up tissues. Tissues make up organs separated according to their functions. For Example, The stomach has interlining of cells, which secretes digestive juices. A middle layer of muscle tissues and an outer covering for protection. So is with the different organs. When we have digestive systems starting from the mouth, tongue, esophagus small and large intestines, the rectum ending in the anus.

The heart receives pure blood from the lungs and pumps it to all organs of the body from where it comes back to the right ventricle of the heart from where it is pumped to the lungs. Blood from the heart reaches the kidneys from where impurities are filtered to become urine for excretion. The brain and the nerves system control all the functions of the body. The muscular skeleton system enables us to move about for our daily functions. The endocrine system is an orchestra of different levels of hormones which makes what we are.

We should not forget that there are separate organs for sight, hearing, smell, taste and touch – eyes, ears, nose, tongue, mouth and skin. Skin and hairs is the outer covering of the body which encloses the different system for the body functions. The skin is the prime organ for temperature regulation in warm blooded animals. Underneath the skin is the fat which is energy stores to future use and also controls temperature.

Disease is caused by bacteria or virus who invades the body. The body is attacked relentlessly, which the body immunity is able to combat. If the organism is virulent or if the body immunity is weak the invaders win and we get diseases requiring medications to help the body to overcome the disease which we call cure. But you should remember that without immunity the body cannot use the medicine as in Aids. A healthy person whose immunity is at peak is free of disease.

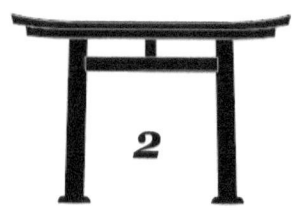

2

Classification -2

Human body according to Ayurvedic system*

Ayurveda is a holistic system of healing which evolved among the sages of ancient India some 3000-5000 years ago. Over the last century, Ayurvedic Medicine has experienced a rebirth and has continued to evolve its holistic approach to health in accordance with modern needs and scientific advances of the day.

1. It focuses on establishing and maintaining balance of the life energies within us, rather than focusing on individual symptoms.
2. It recognizes the unique constitutional differences of all individuals and therefore recommends different regimens for different types of people. Although two people may appear to have the same outward symptoms, their energetic constitutions may be very different and therefore call for very different remedies.
3. Ayurveda is a complete medical system which recognizes that ultimately all intelligence and wisdom flows from one Absolute source. Health manifests by the grace of the Absolute acting through the laws of Nature (Prakriti). Ayurveda assists Nature by promoting harmony between the individual and Nature by living a life of balance according to her laws.
4. Ayurveda describes three fundamental universal energies which regulate all natural processes on both the macrocosmic and microcosmic levels. That is, the same energies which produce effects in the various galaxies and star sys-

tems are operating at the level of the human physiology--in your own physiology. These three universal energies are known as the Tridosha.

5. Finally, the ancient Ayurvedic physicians realized the need for preserving the alliance of the mind and body and offers mankind tools for remembering and nurturing the subtler aspects of our humanity. Ayurveda seeks to heal the fragmentation and disorder of the mind-body complex and restore wholeness and harmony to all people.

Vedas declared that everything in the universe is made up of combinations of the "pancha bhoothams" (Five Elements), Pancha means five, Mahabhoota means basic elements. Human body is a direct replica of the Universe and is also created by it. All physical manifestations in the Universe is created of pancha bhoothams, it is made up of five basic elements. Man is said to be the microcosm and Universe is the macrocosm because what exists in the world exists in man. Man is nothing but a miniature world containing the five elements. These five basic elements are:

1. Akasha (Space),
2. Vayu (Air),
3. Teja (Fire),
4. Jala (Water)
5. Prithvi (Earth).

Man consumes water and food, breathes the air and thus maintains the heat in the body. He is alive on account of the life force given by ether. The earth is the first element which gives fine shape to the body including bones, tissues, muscles, skin, hair etc. Water is the second element representing blood, secretions of the glands, vital fluid etc. Fire is the third element that gives motion, vigor and vitality to the body. It also helps digestion, circulation and simulation besides respiration and the nervous system. Above all, ether is the characteristic of man's mental and spiritual faculties. Ayurvedic masters also found that what Vedas declared is truth. They formed a theory according to this philosophy.

According to Ayurveda every matter is composed of these basic elements in different proportions. The proportion of these decides the state and the properties of the respective matter. Just as human body is made up of these basic elements, every drug that is used as medicine is made up of medicine. Even the three Doshas are said to be composed of these basic pancha bhoothams. For better understanding of these concepts let us consider on the human body the existence of these five basic elements.

- Human body has definite mass: is due to Prithvi
- Human body has definite motion: is due to Vayu
- It contains several structures: space provided for these is due to Akasha
- It shows definite color, brightness and accomplishes digestion: is due to Teja.
- All structure are having strong bonding with each other: is due to Jala

Each Mahabhoota is associated with a special sense.

1. Akasha (Space) - Sense of Hearing
2. Vata - Sense of touch
3. Teja (Fire) - sense of seeing
4. Jala (Water) - Sense of Taste
5. Prithvi (Earth) - Sense of Smell

As mentioned earlier every thing is said to be made of the five basic elements. The three Doshas too have the following composition as far as pancha bhoothams are concerned:

- Vata = Space + Air
- Pitta = Fire + Water
- Kapha = Water + Earth.

Vata Dosha has the mobility and quickness of space and air, which regulates our energies and movements. Pitta Dosha has the metabolic qualities of fire and water; which gives us warmth and perception and the capacity to transform substances within our bodies. Kapha Dosha has the stability and solidity of water and earth, which makes up our structure, our flesh and secretions, and creates solidity and cohesiveness.

Ayurvedic system recognizes Human being to be made of body, mind & soul. Therefore while treating a disease as well; one should keep in mind the whole complex of mind, body and soul and not merely the physical body or the structural organs. The basis of the human body according to Ayurveda depends on three primary factors viz. Dosha (Humors) Dhatu (body tissues) and Malas (excretory products).

Doshas are the functional entities with designated functions. They are also said to be subtle energies. These Doshas are three in number viz., Vata, Pitta and Kapha. Doshas are also called as Humors, which govern or control the functioning of the body. Dhatus are basic body elements which forms body framework and comprise of seven types of body tissues. Malas are excretory waste products that make the body clean and healthy.

Dosha, Dhatu and Malas are the three pillars of body. If any one of these pillars is weak then the healthy state of body falls in a danger. Hence health can also be defined as the perfect equilibrium between Doshas, Dhatus and Malas.

The ancient sages observed that although every individual is constituted of the three Doshas, each of us inherits them in differing proportions. This accounts for our differences in appearance, preferences, aversions, behavioral patterns, and emotional tendencies. The proportion of the three Doshas present in an individual at birth will determine his or her essential constitution or prakriti.

The prakriti remains unchanged during the course of one's lifetime and is genetically determined. It will manifest in us throughout our lifetimes through our physical characteristics, natural urges, likes and dislikes, and psychological predilections as we have stated above. However, one's prakriti will also determine to a great extent how one will develop the highest order of human qualities: love, compassion, and pure consciousness. Thus the proportion of the three Doshas which a person inherits will be at the foundation of his or her experience and existence.

Doshas

The five elements can be seen to exist in the material universe at all scales both organic and inorganic, from peas to planets. When they enter into the biology of a living organism, man for example, they acquire a biological form. This means that the five elements are coded into three biological forces which govern all life processes. These three forces are known as the three Doshas, or simply the tridosha. We can assume that, tridosha. as fundamental biological energies which regulate all the life processes of an individual

When a patient approaches an Ayurvedic Physician, the Physician tries to draw inferences about the status of 3 humors in the individual. Based on his inferences about the Doshas he prescribes medicines. The role of Doshas and their importance in treating an illness and preservation of health is the prime criteria of the physician. The tridosha regulates every physiological and psychological process in the living organism. The interplay among them determines the qualities and conditions of the individual. A harmonious state of the three Doshas creates balance and health; an imbalance, which might be an excess or deficiency, manifests as a sign or symptom of disease.

Vata

It is composed of the elements space and air--the lightest and subtlest of the five elements and is responsible primarily for movements or any type of motion. It is considered in some ways to be the most influential of the three Doshas because it is the moving force behind the other two Doshas, which are incapable of movement without it. If there is any kind of motion present in body, it has been due to presence of Vata Dosha. Blood circulation, movement of food through and through from oral cavity till the excretory product is thrown out is due to Vata, Nerve stimulus, secretion of juices, peristaltic movements are all necessarily attributed to Vata. It is cold in nature.

Pitta

Pitta is directly related with metabolism. Metabolism i.e. conversion of one form of substance in another is necessarily due to Pitta. Think of it as the energy stored in the chemical bonds of all the organic substances which make us up: it is encoded in our hormones, enzymes, organic acids, and neurotransmitters. Pitta is often regarded as the "fire" within the body. Pitta functions in digestion, heat production, providing color to the blood, vision, and skin luster. It is hot in nature.

Kapha

It is the force which provides structure to everything from an individual atom or cell to the sturdy musculoskeletal frame. It is the uniting force. This union can be cell to cell or among the different body parts. It is composed of water and earth. One very important function of Kapha Dosha in the human body is that it governs immunity and resistance against disease; its energy promotes self-healing and the ongoing processes of self-repairs of which we are largely unaware. Where Vata and Pitta effects become active in the body, Kapha acts to limit and control these two forces and prevent their excessive activity. It governs the formation of neuropeptides, stomach linings, and all new cells and tissues of the body which are constantly being destroyed and re-created. It is cold in nature.

The example of Digestive system can help understand the functioning of Doshas in a better way. Vata is related with the movements of stomach, intestines and other parts of alimentary canal as also for the removal of waste products. Pitta is related with the metabolism part that converts food into smaller fractions of carbohydrates, proteins, fats, minerals, and vitamins. Waste product formations like urea, nitrogenous products are also formed due to action of Pitta. Kapha is related with inner mucus lining of the whole alimentary canal starting from the oral cavity and salivary glands. Although these are Doshas are invisible in nature but their presence is felt by fundamental quality (Guna) and their functions (karma). In scientific parlance, Vata comprehends all the phenomena, which comes under the function of the central and sympathetic nervous systems. Pitta consists of the function of thermo genesis and heat production, metabolism within the limits, the process of digestion, coloration of blood, excretion and secretion. Kapha looks after the regulation of the heart and the formation of various glands and structures.

7 Dhatus

The Dhatus or the body tissues in Ayurveda have been described to be of seven types:

1. Shukra Dhatu (reproductive tissues)
2. Majja Dhatu (bone marrow and nervous tissues)
3. Asthi Dhatu (bone)
4. Meda Dhatu (fatty tissues)
5. Mamsa Dhatu (muscle tissues)
6. Rakta Dhatu (formed blood cells)
7. Rasa Dhatu (plasma)

1. Rasa: It is the first basic body tissue. It primarily performs the function of nourishment, giving body energy and glow, soft and smoothness.

2. Rakta: It is an important body element also known as blood.

It gives life to each and every tissue of body.

3. Mamsa: This comprises of the soft and bulky fleshy parts of body. It can be called as muscle tissue and gives strength, gives body a definite shape and structure.

4. Meda: These are soft parts, which are also known as fats or Adipose tissue. It protects the inner structures and acts as reservoir of energy and lubricates the most vital parts such as brain and joints etc.

5. Asthi: The bony tissue that is very hard and solid is what Asthi Dhatu means. It performs the function of protecting vital organs, giving body a definite structure.

6. Majja: Soft, fleshy part situated inside bones also known as Bone marrow is what is termed as Majja Dhatu in Ayurveda. It serves the function of making an individual intelligent and nourishes the bones.

7. Shukra: This refers to a tissue that plays a major role in the reproduction. Although many people try to compare it with Seminal fluid, it is not limited to semen alone. The references suggest that it is some thing, which is circulating through out the body and is responsible for giving bravery like qualities to the individual. May be reproduction of the new cells that is going on every moment forms a part of the functions assigned to Shukra Dhatu. There is no doubt that it is the most important function of Shukra to reproduce by offering the best quality sperms and ovum from both males as well as females.

MALAS (Excretory products)

In every metabolic process there two parts as a result of the process. One is a good and a useful part and the other is waste product. Waste parts or bad products ought to be removed out of body in order to contain their toxic effects on the body. There are two types of Malas viz. Liquid Malas and the Solid Malas. Liquid types of Malas are urine, sweat etc, and solid are stool, hairs, etc.

Health and disease

- All three Doshas are in equilibrium with regard to the individual prakriti
- All seven Dhatus, are in the proper state of strength and integrity
- The digestive fires, Agnis, are balanced resulting in proper appetite, digestion, and assimilation
- The waste materials, Malas, are being produced and eliminated in a regular manner.
- The sense organs, are functioning normally and the mind is undisturbed
- The individual is experiencing happiness and contentment.

The healthy state of all three of these factors is called Samayoga (balanced). However buddhi, senses, and time can also become imbalanced as excessive, deficient, or distorted. These deviations of buddhi, senses, and kala from their normal balanced state are considered in Ayurveda to be the fundamental cause of disease. It is these disharmonies which lead to the vitiation of the doshas, accumulation of ama, weakening of agni, and the entire cascade of the Kriyakala.

Disease manifests as the opposite of some or all of the criteria for health listed above. It is a state of disequilibrium of the Doshas, Dhatus, Agnis, and Malas; the individual is out of harmony both internally and with relation to the environment and experiences unpleasant sensations and misery in some form. The disease state is known as Vikriti, which represents a deviation from that natural proportion of the Doshas. According to Ayurveda, if one lives a natural, simple, and clean life there will always be more momentum in the direction of health than towards disease.

There is an inherent tendency in Nature to move from Vikriti to prakriti and systems of medicine are merely strategies to assist this gentle, yet inexorable, self-healing progression. Ayurveda is indeed the only medical system which describes an elaborate strategy for assessing both the patient and the disease. Ayurveda is stressed more on individual than diseases which is just opposite of allopathic system.

In every patient there is an individual; here treatment is not for organs and symptoms. The astha vaidya or physician is one who is capable of treating eight parts of the body. Hence Ayurveda is holistic treatment which integrates the whole human personality. In every disease condition there is also health. For in actual reality even when a person has a disease of some kind, he or she has certainly not lost his or her entire health. Aspects of health always remain with a person along side the disease state. This important reservoir of health is the foundation of his eventual recovery according to the principle of svabhavoparamavada--the tendency for the body to eliminate the root of a disease and to heal itself when properly supported.

Note – Taken from various Internet sources..

Medicine

All our foods are medicines. We live our lives mainly due to the food we eat. Hence every food has a medicinal value. Normally in our daily life we have a combination of food. Such a combination of food is consumed while we are healthy. We have to change this combination (or add or less from it) while we have diseases. While we have sickness we have to consume other combination of food along with normal diet. There are different combinations of food as per different diseases. This is according to the Doshas, Dhatus and digestive natures of the sick.

Each person has to be given a particular type of food (medicine), which is a combination of plants roots, leaves or fruits. We cannot see any plant in the universe, which does not have a medicinal value. Ayurvedic saints after immense research distinguished each plant and found their value in healing and prescribed it as food as per sickness. Not just plants, all living creatures, animate and inanimate objects too posses a value. The Saints found all these and prescribed them in a combination (or alone) to particular diseases. When this combination of food is consumed, then the diseases will get healed. Mostly for diseases related to Vata, medicine should be taken along with oil, when it is Pita then medicine should be taken with ghee and for Kapha the medicine is taken with honey.

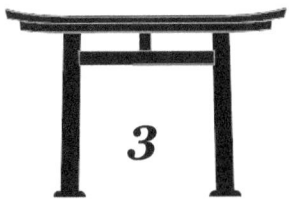

3   *Subtle Bodies*

Aura

Modern science tells us that the human organism is not just a physical structure made of molecules; but like everything else, is composed of energy fields. We are constantly changing, ebbing, and flowing, just like the sea. We are constantly swimming in a vast sea of life energy fields, thought fields, and Bioplasmic forms, moving about and streaming off the body. We are vibrating; radiating Bioplasma itself. Scientists are learning to measure these subtle changes.

Every body emits a network of subtle energies invisible to the naked eye. These energies appear in several high frequency layers around the body. The frequency of these energies increases with every layer. Throughout history, this external energy field or matrix is called the as the aura, corona, halo, and more recently the human bioelectrical energy field, or Bioplasma. It extends about 10 to 12 inches from the body. It expands dramatically during Reiki attunement. After four attunement Aura can be expanded from 7 to 9 feet, permanently. Transformation on spiritual level is reflected in the expansion of Aura. Inanimate object also have an Aura. Most personnel objects draw energy of the owner and radiate this energy. Gems, crystals etc show interesting Auras with many layers and complicated patterns that can be used in healing. We can see aura through Kirlian photography.

Seven layers of Aura

1. Etheric body
2. Emotional body
3. Mental body
4. Astral body
5. Template body
6. Celestial body
7. Ketharic or Casual body

Auras and diseases

Through Aura meters, Aura cameras and also by clairvoyants, a disease can be seen in the energy body even before it manifests itself on the visible physical body. Non-clairvoyants may scan or feel that the inner Aura of the affected part is either smaller or bigger than usual. For instance, before a person suffers from cough and colds, the bio-plasmic throat and lungs are "Pranically" depleted and can be observed clairvoyantly as grayish. These areas when scanned can be felt as hollows in the inner Aura.

Another example: A person who is about to suffer from jaundice can be observed clairvoyantly as having a gray solar plexus and liver. Physical tests or diagnoses will show the patient as normal or healthy. Unless the patient is treated, the disease will manifest inevitably on the visible physical body with out much delay.

The Chakras

Quantum physics tells us that material substances are composed not only of observable matter, but also more subtle field components with organized energy patterns, boundaries and definitions.

The physical body is composed of solids, liquids, and gases, including such parts as the bones, blood system, nervous system, brain and endocrine glands. The chakras, naadis and auras the subtle bodies. The true seats of the seven main chakras are in the ethereal body. Each chakra is like a solid ball of energy inter-penetrating the physical body, in the same way that a magnetic field can interpenetrates the physical body. The word chakra is derived from the Sanskrit word meaning "wheel" or "vortex".

The junctions of Naadis with Sushumna Naadi are known as Chakras, subtle centers of vital energy. Chakras are situated in various points of Sushumna (spinal cord). They are all supported by the vertebral column; the five regions of the spinal column (coccygeal, sacrum, lumbar, dorsal and cervical region) correspond with the regions of the five Chakra: Muladharam, Swadhistanam, Manipurakam, Anahatam and Vishudhi. The Chakras are centers of Pranashakti, the cosmic energy in latent shape. Prana has two types. The Subtle or vital is called Sukshumam and the gross is called Sthoolam .Subtle Prana moves in the nervous system of the subtle body(chakras, naadis, auras). Physical Prana moves in the nervous system of the gross physical body.

The scientific explanation of chakras is; Within every living body, although on the subtle rather than the gross or the physical level, there are said to be a series of energy fields or centers of consciousness, which in traditional Tantric teachings are called chakras [1](Wheels), or, [2] padmas (Lotuses). They are said to be located either along, or just in front of, the backbone, even though they might express themselves externally at points along the front of the body (navel, heart, throat, etc). Associated with the chakras is a latent subtle energy, called Kundalini in Shaktism, and Tumo in Tibetan Buddhist Tantra.

The chakras are more denser than the auras, but not as dense as the physical body, but they interact with the physical body through two major vehicles, the endocrine system and the nervous system. Each of the seven chakras is associated with one of the seven endocrine glands, and also with a particular group of nerves called a plexus. Thus, each chakra can be associated with particular parts of the body and particular functions within the body controlled by that plexus or that endocrine gland associated with that chakra.

Chakras and diseases

Each Chakra is designed to supervise and maintain the perfect operation of the bodily systems under its control. This purification is done by spinning in pure or positive vibrations and spinning out impure or negative ones. Chakras are blocked by gross negativity accumulated by years of neglect or self-destructive activities like drugs, drinking, violence, anger, hatred, fanaticism, sexual deviation and so on. When chakras start to heal we get immediate benefits; small anxieties decrease and some joy and objectivity begins to manifest, and the blocked Chakras begin to rotate properly again. The patient's chakras receive the energy, which serves to vitalize his physical body and more especially his endocrine gland system, thereby bringing about physical health.

Seven chakras

1. Muladharam(root chakra)- (mula = root; hadaram = support)

It is located at the base of the spine or the coccyx area. This controls, energizes and strengths the whole visible physical body, especially the spine, the production and the quality of blood produced, the tissues of the body, the internal and sexual organs. People with highly activated basic chakra are usually healthy.

Diseases: Excretory, Immunity, Sciatica, Varicose Veins, Rectal tumors/cancer, Depression, Immune-related disorder

2. *Swadhistanam (spleen chakra) - (swa = vital force; adishthanam = seat).*

It is located on the navel and it affects the general vitality of a person. It controls fluid functions of the body, and energizes the sexual organs and the spleen. The spleen purifies the blood of disease-causing germs. It also destroys worn-out blood cells.

Diseases: Reproductive disorders; pre-menstrual tensions and irregular periods, Sexual impotency, constipation, chronic lower back pain, Urinary problems appendicitis, low vitality and other intestine related diseases.

3. *Manipurakam(solar plexus chakra)- (mani = gem, purakam = city)*

It is located on the left part of the abdomen between the front solar plexus chakra and the naval chakra ("Naabhi"). Digestion of food is an important function. It controls and energizes the diaphragm, pancreas, liver, stomach and to a certain extent energizes the large and small intestines, appendix, lungs, heart and other parts of the body.

Diseases: Repressed energy at cell level, often leading to cancer; arthritis, problems with the above organs ('butterflies', constipation, diarrhea, ulcers, digestive problems); migraines, Kidney disease, diabetes, ulcer, hepatitis, heart disease in relation to our fear of power

4. *Anahatam (heart chakra) – (Anahatam = unbeaten)*

It lies behind heart and energizes and controls the Love & compassion, command on all organs by circulatory system, function of the heart and lungs and higher emotions.

Diseases: Heart attack; problems with blood pressure, problems of the circulatory system, immune system disease (AIDS), Hypertension, Bronchial pneumonia, Allergies, lung problems such as asthma, tuberculosis, and others.

5. Vishudhi(throat chakra) – (Vishudhi = pure)

It is located at the center of the throat. It controls and energizes the throat and the lymphatic system.

Diseases: mainly of the throat and lungs, such as, throat cancer, sore throat, all are related to throat chakra.

6. Aagnya(third eye chakra) - (Aagnya= command or permission)

It is located at the area between the eyebrows. It controls and energizes the brain to a certain extent and the nervous system.

Diseases: mainly of the autonomic nervous system; hormonal imbalance; headaches; migraines; sinusitis; Brain tumor, dizziness; depression; eye/ear problems, loss of memory, paralysis and epilepsy.

7. Sahasraram (crown chakra) - (Sahasraram= 1000 petals)

It lies at the top of the head and controls and energizes the brain and the entire body. It is also one of the major entry points of Prana into the body. It is the spiritual headquarters of the body.

Diseases: Serious psychotic disorders; Central nervous system, Energetic disorders, Mystical depression, Chronic exhaustion that is not linked to a physical disorder, Extreme sensitivity to light, sound, etc.

Note – Taken from various Internet sources

Naadis

In electrical engineering, it is an established principle that all electrical currents moving through a wire produce surrounding electromagnetic fields. Accordingly, when our psychological and emotional energies are sent throughout the body as electrical impulses along the biological (neural) and energy (meridian) pathways, these transmissions cause electromagnetic fields to radiate outside the body. By this process, the tangible features (frequency, waveform, etc.) of these radiating electrical field energies are characteristic of the mental activity that generated them, as much research in this field has revealed.

The Sanskrit term Naadi comes from the root Naadi that means "motion". It is like a tubular organ of the astral body through which the Prana (vital force) flows. There are 101 main naadis in the human body and altogether 72,000 naadis spread through out the body. They are the subtle bodies in the human body just like the nervous system. It is filled with rasas (hormones). Vital energy force circulates through it. Nadis are the equivalent to our blood vessels but instead of transporting blood it transports energy.

The naadis are known as meridian points in the acupuncture. The most important among the main Nadis are Ida, Pingla and Sushumna. If there is any block in these passages that part will be affected and disease occurs in that part. This block can be removed by passing the energy through that. In acupressure theory they say the Ida and Pingla as yin and yang. When the yin and yang are balanced, the living system exhibits physical health; when they are unbalanced, it become diseased. Imbalance of yang results in excessive organic activity while the imbalance in yin brings insufficient functioning. Both of these imbalances end up as physical illness. The ancient art of acupuncture and acupressure focuses on balancing the yin and the yang.

12 primary meridians

There are two systems of channels or meridians, namely primary and secondary meridians. Primary meridians pass through internal organs but secondary do not. There are 12 pairs of primary meridians with Chi flowing in continuous circulation through the following organs: lungs, colon, stomach, spleen, heart, intestines, urinary bladder, kidneys, pericardium, triple warmer, gall bladder and liver. These primary meridian points are mainly used in healing.

Reiki and the meridians

A Reiki treatment will balance the yin and yang or Ida and Pingla and facilitate a smooth flow of vital energy through the naadis. Reiki can dissolve blockages in meridians and helps to restore the body's healthy flow of Chi.

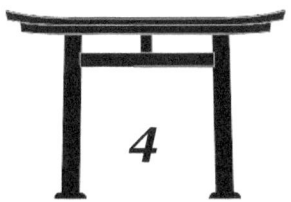

4   **Attunement**

There is an attunement procedure similar like in the first level but the major difference is, the symbols are attached with this attunement. This technique was not there in the first level. The availability of symbols to the students makes them a complete Reiki channel.

Attunement and chakras

All attunements are done to open the chakras. Awakening of the chakras enables the power of healing. First level attunements will have an impact on Aura also. In the physical body, it facilitates the metabolism with increased divine and Vital Energy, which have the power to heal yourself or others. This holy attunement brings the divine association between the disciple and the Energy. It is the sacred thread, which connects us with the inner energy and outer energy for the first time.

The first-level initiation involves four attunements designed to step up the vibration rates to the Sahasraram, Aagnya, Vishudhi. and Anahatam. Our body has major and minor chakras. The chakra in the palm is a minor chakra. The palm chakra opens up in the attunement. The divine connection obtained will rapidly get in touch with the palm chakras. Through the palm chakra the energy is given to the patient.

There is only one empowerment in the second-level. If the disciple had taken first level empowerment from a different master then he has to give re-empowerment for the first level then only they are eligible for the second level. This procedure is mainly followed because; each empowerment works along with the frequency of the previous one.

All masters follow different procedures in the empowerment and also their frequency levels are also different. Hence the continuity of the empowerment levels differs and this will have an impact in the empowerment. The empowerment will be incomplete and also the disciples will not be fully aligned with lineage of the new master. Hence they are given the re-empowerment to bestowal the new level without breaking its link and to acquire its full benefits.

This is also the same procedure if you take the master level from a different master. He has to undergo the re-empowerment of the first and second level. You are blossoming with each empowerment, so they expand the conduit of the previous level and enhance the capability of extracting the energy. Second level empowerment activates the three symbols (second-level). The Ajna chakra is opened up to its double capacity than in first level empowerments, which will improve the intuition. Sahasrara and Anahata will also have an impact. It triggers the healing on all four levels.

The third-level empowerment activates the master symbol, which enhances Reiki's power by a factor of eight. You are empowered with the two master symbols in this level.

Interpreting sensations of hands in Reiki

After the second degree Reiki, the healer will start to feel some sensations in the hand while treating others or in self-treatments. The sensation will keep changing with levels or higher attunement. In the first degree most people feel a warmth sensation. In the second degree they complain that they are not getting that much warmth like in the first degree and they even think that they have even lost their healing ability with the attunement of the second degree. The fact is Reiki does not depend upon warmth or chilled.

If you are actually a good healer your hand will be according to the situations, for example if the patient's body is warm then your hands will feel chilled, when the patients body is cold, then your hands will feel the warmth, all these will come only after many healing experiences. Again there will be progress after the master degree or the nature of the sensation will be changed. It is because Reiki sensation will change according to the different imbalances in the same body. It is the highest stage in healing when our hands will feel one thing while person will feel the opposite.

The most common experiences of healer's are:

1. A feeling of warmth in the hands.
2. Tingling or pulsing up or down the arms and in the body.
3. Chilled or cool energy running through the hands.
4. The cessation of mental talk, and increased calm.
5. Deep relaxation.
6. Visual impressions, seeing colors, lights or images.
7. Hands feeling drawn to particular areas.
8. Hands feeling repelled from particular areas.
9. Hands feeling like they are stuck or glued in an area.
10. Hands feeling like they are a few inches inside the area that is being worked on.
11. An occasional sharp or dull pain in your hands or arms.
12. A slight vibration in the hands or arms.

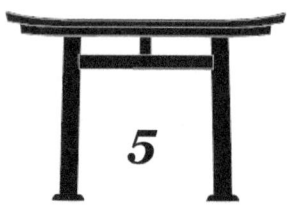

5   History of Symbols

There is still higher order of formal worship- the world of symbolism. The forms are still there, but they are neither trees nor stone nor images nor relics of saints. They are symbols. The circle is a great symbol of eternity. There is a square; the well-known symbol cross; and two figures like S and Z crossing each other.

Swami Vivekananda

Most of the symbols are derived from the religion. It is mainly because the symbols are worshiped in religion for thousands of years; hence it should have a value. Those, which are worshiped for thousands of years, must have a value other wise how it was followed by millions? Truth is the only thing, which does not have any change; all else is subject to change. These symbols are still in worship hence these symbols are true. All the traditional symbols are derived from other sources in Japanese culture, and can be found in their spiritual books or temples. However, they may not have had any energy associated with them (or perhaps a different type of energy) in their original form. In fact, several are not symbols but Japanese phrases.

Symbols have actually been created from Japanese Kanji which means they are simply words from the Japanese language. Their names can be found in a Japanese/English dictionary. The first two symbols vary from this somewhat. While the names of the Power and Mental/Emotional symbols are Japanese, the symbols themselves may be shamanic or a combination of Sanskrit and Japanese kanji. It is a practice of

Japanese Buddhists' to sometimes combine ancient Sanskrit with Japanese kanji in their sacred writings and symbols so the way these first two symbols are drawn may have been influenced by this practice. The distant and Master symbols are completely Japanese kanji, both in their names and in the way they are drawn and all the characters can be found in a Japanese/English dictionary.

It is interesting to note that the name of the Usui Master symbol can be found in "The Encyclopedia of Eastern Philosophy and Religion" and is translated to mean "treasure house of the great beaming light." It is said to be, "a Zen expression for one's own true nature or Buddha-nature of which one becomes cognizant in the experience of enlightenment or Satori." This is quite a profound definition. Perhaps it is called the Master symbol because it gives us direct connection to the Master within which is the real source of Reiki. Also, since the Usui Master symbol is a powerful symbol from Zen Buddhism, one wonders how much help Dr. Usui received from the Zen Buddhists or other Japanese religious groups when he rediscovered Reiki.

The above information indicates that the Usui Reiki symbols are not exclusive to Usui Reiki. They existed prior to Dr. Usui's use of them. Also, because they are Japanese, it is not likely that he discovered them in a Sanskrit sutra as some have thought. It is much more likely that Dr. Usui received the symbols in his mystical experience on Mt. Kurama, (located just north of Kyoto) or that he had prior knowledge of them from the Zen Buddhists or other religious groups he had studied with. Since the symbols are Japanese and we know that the Master symbol is from Zen Buddhism, perhaps the sutra in which he discovered the formula for healing was Zen Buddhist rather than a Sanskrit sutra. (Even though there is a Sanskrit sutra that contains a formula for healing.) In addition, the Usui Master symbol also appears as part of the symbol on the Goshintai, which is the sacred scroll of the Johrei Fellowship.

There is also another argument that Usui taught symbols to a very small number of people, just in the last few years of his life. The vast majority of his students were taught in a very different way. Most of his students were given meditations to use so that they could, over a long period of time, become more and more familiar with the three energies taught at second-degree level, for example. Once they were thoroughly familiar with the energies, once they had *become* the energies again and again, then they were given a shortcut - a trigger - to connect them to those energies. The triggers that they used were ancient Shinto mantras called kotodama, or jumon, not symbols.

In the August 1999, Japanese Reiki Master Horoshi Doi explained that the "symbols" were first introduced by Usui-sensei as a form of training wheels for some students. Sensei discovered that some students were unable to accept that the energies they received beyond the Reiki energy could be transmitted just by will. And so to assist one student with distant Reiki, he had the person focus on an old Buddhist mantra, which Dr. Hayashi came to teach as the Connection energy. This eventually spread to the other 3 main energies shared by Sensei as well. Sensei obviously drew on his previous research in order to provide an appropriate mantra or symbol. In Dr. Hayashi's more structured form of Reiki, Usui Shiki Ryoho (Usui Method of Healing), the use of the symbols seemed to become solidified into a standard part of the training, and if at any point they were later de-emphasized, this was not passed on by Mrs. Takata in the west. Thus the symbols grew in importance along side the energy they convey.

*Research about the Origin of the Symbols**

Note: Research on the origin of the Reiki symbols is continuing and this information will continue to develop. Hence all the information's are incomplete.

We cannot trace the origins of symbols. Some says that Usui Sensei got it from sacred texts of Indian and Buddhist origin. Others says that he got the symbols from the temple of Kuruma Yama in the mountain where he mediated for 21 days. There is also an argument that symbols are obtained from vision. Some even says that there was no symbol in the Usui times. He used other techniques such as Kotadama, Hasturi-ho etc. before reaching the death Usui created symbols for Western disciples such as Hayashi. Again it is getting more confused. One thing is sure there was symbols existed in the Usui era and he may or may not utilize it. The symbols have got tremendous powers, which are proven without doubt. Hence we can say that symbol definitely works and we can erase our doubts about the origin from our intellect.

Still it is interesting to know about the origins. It can be termed only as a curiosity. In research conducted by scholars, particularly Mr. Arjava Peter states that, the actual word Reiki is not a household term in Japan. It comes from an ancient Shinto's mantra to protect one who chants it. So Word Reiki as such is a symbol (for protection) this mantra has been passed from Shinto teacher to student by word of mouth for centuries and we are initiated to it only after we promised not to pass it on to any one. Symbols appear both in Shintoism and ancient Buddhism. CKR, TM and SHK are slight variations from the originals. The pronunciation is Japanese. These symbols came from India to Tibet and from there to China and Japan. HSZSN is derived from several Kanji and DKM is an original Kanji. Kanji is a Japanese word that was brought from China to Japan long ago.

The DKM is used at the Kurama temple (where Usui did his 21 day Lotus Repentance Meditation and had Satotri and discovered Reiki). The DKM as used in the Kurama temple is to represent "Sonten". For the Kurama-Kokyo, the deities Mao-son, Bishamon-ten, and Senju-Kannon [or Senju-Kanzeon] are seen as symbols of the universal soul, forming the triune deity which they call: 'Sonten'. Mao-son is seen as representing the power of Sonten, Bishamon-ten is seen as representing the light of Sonten, and Senju-Kannon - the love of Sonten. There are some sects in Japan that believe that all the Buddha's have emerged in/as/of Sonten.

And when they discover that the term DKM is sometimes applied to Sonten. Sonten is the "Living or Supreme Soul of the universe". Sonten is "Glorious Light" or Great Shining Light this is what the DKM represents. 'DKM refers to the 'great illuminating wisdom' of deity - and can be properly applied to each and every Butsu.

It seems there is a connection between the symbolic meanings of the shuji of Mao-son (in Japanese: 'un', Sanscrit: 'hum') and the CKR. The symbol has got a slight resemblances of CKR.

Mao-son 'un'.

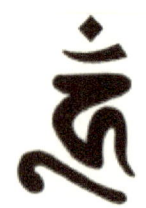

In Japanese Esoteric Buddhism, each deity (Buddha, Bodhisattva, Myo-o, etc) - and each of the Five Elements - has its associated symbol - known as a shuji ('seed' character): a particular character from the 'Siddham' form of the Sanskrit script. In Sanskrit, this character is called 'Hrih'. Beyond its meditative use, the sacred Siddham script (brought to Japan in the 9thC) is employed by Mikkyo Buddhists exclusively for writing mantras, sutras and magical-religious Tantric formulas.

This shuji is held to be the 'sacred sign' of the given deity, and is regarded as itself possessing the divine grace and power of that deity. Amongst other things, a deity's shuji is essentially perceived as a single-character depiction of the sacred mantra of the deity, and as such invokes the merit associated with the recital/repetition of that mantra. We can assume a meaning from the above, shuji is the Beeja Akshram in Sanskrit. All devas have a Beeja Akshram and is the mantra of that Deva. When it is chanted it helps the chanter.

SHK ('Spiritual Composure') is almost certainly a stylized form of the Siddham character Kiriku (pronounced: k'rik). Kiriku is the 'sacred sign' of Amida Butsu (or Amida

Nyorai as he is called in Mikkyo Buddhist traditions), and is regarded as itself possessing the divine grace of Amida. 'Mariko Obaasan' - a Buddhist Nun said to have known Usui Sensei, claims that he was a devotee of Amida - and that he made an offering to Amida every day.

Amida - Buddha of Infinite Light & Life - is widely worshipped in various schools of Japanese Buddhism, including Tendai. He is the main deity in Jodo (Pure Land) Buddhism; and also in Jodo Shin (True Pure Land) Buddhism which holds that Spiritual Peace of Mind and salvation are to be achieved by relying on his power. [Usui Sensei's Memorial and family tomb is in a Jodo Shin temple cemetery].The sacred mantra of Amida: "Namu Amida Butsu", and as such invokes

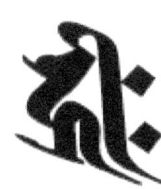 the merit associated with the recital/repetition of that mantra, thus bringing Spiritual Peace of Mind ('Spiritual Composure') to the individual reciting the mantra, or to any other being to whom the recites chooses to 'transfer' this merit. The symbol of Amida has got slight resemblances of SHK. The meaning of the sacred mantra of Amida is given to the meaning of SHK.

The HSZSN 'symbol' is technically not a 'symbol' per se, but rather is a stylized combination of five kanji, and therefore, is simply the phrase: H S Z S N, written in Japanese. Just as calligraphers in the West - when writing a phrase in the Roman Alphabet - will frequently embellish their artwork with flourishes and overlaps, and often combine letters or allow them to run into one-another, this is also the case with Japanese kanji calligraphy. HSZSN mantra [or: Nen Shingon* as it is sometimes called] is essentially a call to 'Mindfulness' - it reminds us of the 7th step in the Noble 8-Fold Path of Buddhism.

*Source James Deacon

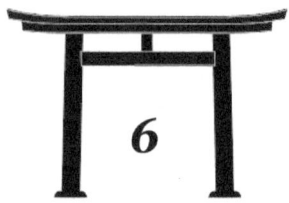

6   **Reiki Symbols**

1. The 'Power' symbol (CKR)

Translation: I command the universal energy.
Takata-Sensei translated CKR as 'put the [spiritual] power here'.

We assume that 'all the powers in the universe are here'. This means that the greater powers in the universe may have a resonance with this symbol. Through this symbol the Reiki practitioner is getting connected to the source from where the power of vibration originated.

Writing of the symbol according to James Deacon

The term 'CKR', when written in one particular set of kanji (Japanese ideograms): 勅令 refers to an Imperial Edict, Proclamation or Order ("by command of the Emperor"). Written in a different set of kanji: 直霊 it can be conceptually translated as something like: 'In the presence of the spirits(kami)'. according to some theories, associated with honji suijaku.

[This is one reason some people consider the symbol to be of Shinto origin.] It has, on a number of occasions, been suggested that the CKR represents a coiled snake with it's head raised (A doctrine of Shinto-Buddhist syncretism), the real forms of kami are actually snakes.

2. The 'Emotional Healing' symbol (SHK)

Translation: I have the key.

We assume that 'the formula for mental peace'. This symbol contains powerful and pacifying vibrations to attain mental and emotional peace. Through this symbol the Reiki practitioner is getting connected to the source from where mind by itself shines in calm.

Writing of the symbol according to James Deacon

As to the actual phrase; 'SHK' - we have to remember that this [as is the case with CKR] is simply a transliteration of the Japanese, and just as in English where (for example) the words 'rite', 'write' and 'right' all have the same sound, so too in Japanese there are often many words that sound the same, yet are written in different kanji and have very different meanings. There has often been debate over the transliteration of both CKR and SHK.

SHK refers to disposition; inclination; characteristic; idiosyncrasy. It can also refer to emotional calmness or unconcern. (S here implies: emotion; feelings; passion. H K = calmness; composure; unconcern.)

When written as: 聖平気 S implies something Spiritual, Holy or Sacred. Again, H&K = calmness; composure; unconcern - thus implying: 'Spiritual Composure' - the perfect antidote for mental-emotional dis-order.

3. The 'Distant' symbol (HSZSN)

Translation: The Buddha in me sees the Buddha in you.

Hiroshi Doi interprets HSZSN as: Right consciousness is the root for everything. Another interpretation is: Correct Thought (Mindfulness) is the essence of being.

From my viewpoint, it has got the meaning of Vedanta that your soul is the same as my soul. Thus the meaning is, "May the Prana in me which is the same in you, connect ourselves for harmony and peace or enhance the well being". Thus by helping others I am helping myself. The symbol has got the vibration that can travel to any corner of the world and the subtle bodies. Through this symbol the Reiki practitioner is getting connected to the source from where is beyond time and space or above our human intellect.

Writing of the symbol according to James Deacon

H 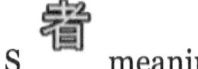 meaning -root, source, origin, essence, basis, counter for long things, book, present, main, true or real.

S meaning- someone or person.

Z meaning- just so, this, right, just or proper.

S meaning- correct, justice, certainly, exactly or righteous.

N meaning- mindfulness, wish, sense, idea, thought, feeling, desire, attention or concern.

Non-Traditional Symbols

Some Reiki schools have added other symbols than these three in their Reiki practice. The Symbols are tools for healing. All the symbols other than Reiki symbols are known as non- traditional symbols. There is no need to add other symbols, because Reiki symbols have all the powers to heal. Since there is no end for extracting energy or the knowledge about healing hence, different symbols are handy. These non-traditional symbols are obtained through the clairvoyants of different masters or from sacred texts.

Non-traditional symbols will not work without charging it with the Reiki symbols, so these symbols will get the quality of that symbol plus the quality of Reiki symbols. You can also use any symbols, which is obtained to you from clairvoyance.

Draw the non-traditional symbol in your hands then draw CKR. This process charges the non-traditional symbols with a powerful energy, which was absent before. Personally, I never use any non-traditional symbols for healing.

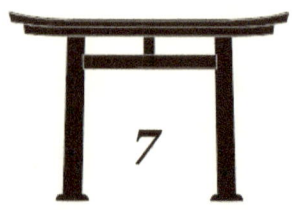

7   Treatment Procedure

All diseases can be classified as:

1. Acute diseases
2. Chronic diseases

1. Acute diseases

All diseases, which occur and disappear in a short period, are labeled as acute diseases. They are diseases, which are common or temporary. The common cold, influenza, fever, headache, dysentery, minor injuries, constipation, and tooth-ache are all examples of diseases, which fall under this category. They are not considered serious diseases. However, some of the diseases mentioned above may or may not be considered the starting point of serious diseases. If the diagnosed symptoms do not develop into serious diseases then they fall in the acute category which can be treated successfully during a short period by almost all types of medical systems such as Modern medicine, Ayurveda, and Homeopathy, Siddha, Unani, etc.

2. Chronic diseases

All ailments, which have a serious or fearful nature, are classified as Chronic Diseases, Which can even be fatal in time. Such ailments should be treated over a long period by all medical systems. Ailments such as Cancer, AIDS, Heart Attack, Diabetics, Blood Pressure, kidney Stones, Viral Infections, Migraines, Psoriasis, Arthritis, Chronic Back Pain, and Tuberculosis are categorized as Chronic Diseases.

Different types of medical systems can treat a few among these successfully. Complete recovery is a dilemma for the vast majority of diseases, or most of the identified medical systems are ineffective to treat many such chronic maladies. One such effective healing proven to effectively cure such trauma is known as Holistic Medicine which has an important role, either by supporting or curing these life- threatening maladies.

Healing crisis

Healing crisis is the period where the body releases the toxins. It is the cleansing period of the body. During this period there will be an unpleasant feeling or an ill feeling. All the unpleasant feelings or ailments during the cleansing period are called as healing crisis. The body's first attempt to achieve health may in some cases be experienced as momentarily increased pain in already damaged areas or in areas with chronic pain. This pain normally lasts only a short period, and it is a good sign that the injury or problem is actively healing. However, in a few cases the pain has been known to last for as long as up to a year.

In short we can say healing crisis is the corrective period of the body. It is a temporary stage before complete healing. Diseases are aggravated while healing. The body itself projects the crisis. The solution for healing crisis is to give Reiki to the water and drink it to compensate for the amount of toxins re- moved from the body. The toxins will be oozed out as cold, cough, dysentery, fever etc. We cannot get any prior idea of what type of healing crisis may occur for the energy receiver. The indication of pain or weariness may increase. Constipation may occur. Sleeping will be disturbed. Asthma problems may increase and sometimes-even oxygen cylinders must be used.

Anything can happen in the healing crisis except death. In some cases there will be no healing crisis. An example for no healing crisis is those related to the heart. In such cases healing crisis are seen utmost rarely. Showing patience in these adverse conditions of healing crisis is the main remedy. Give maximum Reiki during the crisis and do not feel afraid or lazy. Do not think of the healing crisis as bad. Everything is beneficial and works toward a positive outlook.

Can diseases pass over to the healer?

There are lesser chances to obtain the diseases of the patient to the healer, which is most common in energy healings. The main difference between Reiki and other modes of treatments where "Prana" is used for healing, is the initiation. For example the Pranic healing treatment founded by "Chok sui" has no initiation. By studying the book one can become a healer and there is no initiation for them. Initiation is the key for healing. It bestows the ability to heal by opening the chakras. When this chakra is opened up then we will get tremendous power for healing, creativity and other extra ordinary abilities. Thus only by an initiation the practitioner is getting the power to heal, which is not obtained by book reading or by a lecture. This qualification to heal via initiation is absent in other forms of energy healing treatment that is why diseases are transmitted. If you are not qualified for doing something then it's de-merit will also bind you.

Symbols are the other unique aspects of the Reiki, which excels the other healing modalities. First initiation and then the symbols are the two major protective pillars of Reiki, which gives the healer the safety from obtaining the diseases from the patient. When we heal automatically there will be doubts in mind about the safety or there will be negative thought forms in the mind. This thought forms does not have the capability to transfer the diseases because of the protective power of the symbols and the intellect of Reiki. Reiki has its own intellect it will not have a negative impact on both, the healer as well as the patient.

There is no evidence that the healer will obtain the diseases of the patient in Reiki treatments. The diseases of the patient will no way affect the healer but on some occasions it can create a temporary imbalance in the healer, which will be gone by self-treatment or meditation after some time.

Quick treatment for patients

If you do not have the time to do a full body treatment you can do a quick treatment. Quick treatment given to acute disease is different from chronic one. In acute diseases treating only the diseased area is sufficient while in chronic diseases it is necessary to do whole body treatment. It is quite common that smaller problems like headaches and different aches and pains disappear within a short period of treatment; this will boost your confidence before you treat chronic diseases.

When giving short treatment you should clearly differentiate between a short treatment and a full body treatment. If you are going to give a few minutes of Reiki, then explain that this to the patient that it is not a complete treatment; it will offer only temporary relief. And to cure completely systematic treatment is needed.

However at times quick treatment method is affective for chronic patients also. Following is a way to do quick treatment to such patients. The quick treatment means giving treatment only to the chakra positions. There is also another procedure that is to treat the four head positions and the throat positions. Treating the head is an important method. All the meridian points have the roots at head. By treating the head all the body gets energy. Treating head position and then treat the diseased organ is also a better way of quick treatments.

Positions for quick treatment: there are two methods, one by putting two hands on the same chakra while the other, is putting one hand on one chakra and the other hand on the next chakra. First method is listed below.

1. One hand on the forehead, the other at the back.
2. One hand on the front of throat, the other at the back.
3. One hand on the front of the heart, the other at the back.
4. One hand on the front of the solar plexus, the other at the

back,

5. One hand on the front of the spleen, the other at the back.
6. One hand on the front of the genitals, and the other at the back.
7. One hand under the left sole, the other under the right.

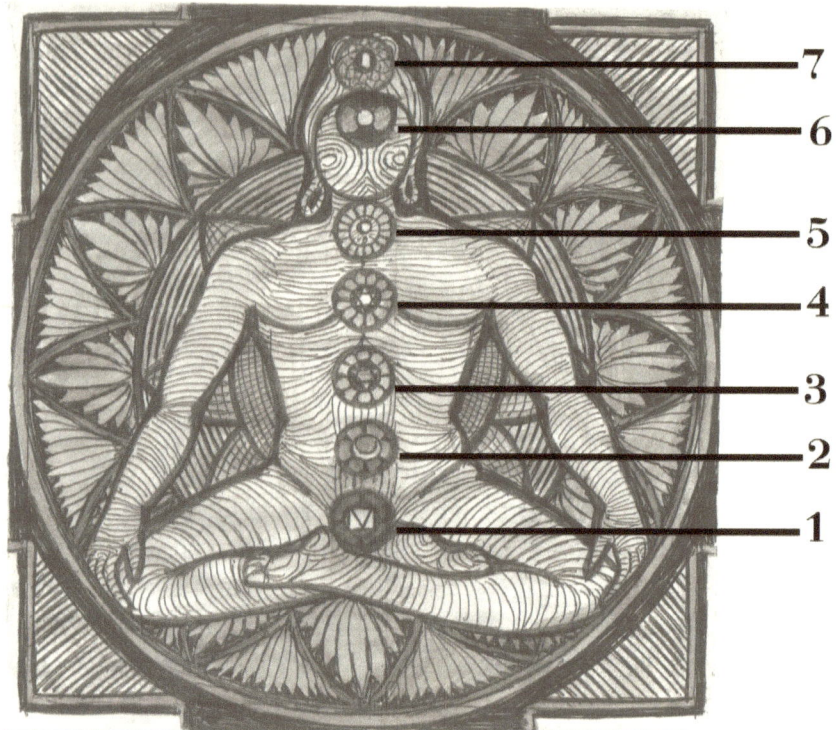

1.BASE CHAKRA-MULADHARAM.
2.HARA CHAKRA-SWADHISTANAM.
3.SOLAR PLEXUS CHAKRA-MANIPURAKAM.
4.HEART CHAKRA-ANAHATHAM.
5.THROAT CHAKRA-VISHUDHI.
6.BROW CHAKRA-AAGNYA.
7.CROWN CHAKRA-SAHASRARAM.

Procedure for the treatment.

1. Reiki prayer before and after the sessions.
2. Draw all the symbols in the hand and chant their names.
3. Stroke and seal the patient after the treatment.

You should never forget these three things in a session. The normal procedure in a Reiki treatment:

First thing is to clear the negative energy in the room by drawing a big CKR in the room and treatment bed either by hand or by stick (which used to smudge). Then protect your self with the stick by smudging the aura by CKR. Then smudge the aura of the patient with CKR. Ask him to lay comfortably in the bed with eyes closed or open. Ask him to relax the body and mind. Play soft or devotional music in a reasonable sound. Draw CKR in your hand and sweep the negative energy of the patient.

If it is chronic case salt water should be used. Sweep the right side of the body and then sweep the left side. When using the salt-water sweep the right side of the body first and start with the left when you reach the ribs of the body then move the hand in the direction of right leg and sweep through that direction. Never sweep the left leg with the salt water. While doing it with salt water one time sweep is enough but you can do more if needed. If you are not using salt water then sweep till you feel the negative energy is removed.

After that give a little energy in the aura. Let the negative energy be replaced with the positive energy. Then go and wash your hands. Washing hands after the sweeping is to remove the negative energy from the hands. This is the first phase in the treatment. Only on the first few days (three days) this procedure is required but you can continue if you think so.

Draw all the three symbols in order in your hand and chant their names respectively. Withdraw your ego from the treatment and ask the Divine energy to guide you till the end of the treatment. Place your hands on the eyes (first position) and begin the treatment. Concentrate your mind or chant mantra in mind during the treatment. Watch closely the sensations and act according to it. Never speak while you treat.

Remember hand positions are not important and move hands on all parts of the body and give energy where it is needed. Means, Use symbols on all are parts, which you think is needed. Symbols will increase the flow of energy. Draw symbols if you have lack of concentration. If you are not in a mood to treat then draw symbols on all the parts of the body. Treat the head firstly. Usui considered all the five positions in the head as equal to full body treatment. Treat the front side of the body and backside after that.

If you finished treating the whole body, first do stroke. Stroke means drawing three lines with three fingers (2,3and 4th finger) from crown chakra to root chakra. It is better to draw from root chakra to crown chakra. Do it three times. After that feel in mind that energy is balanced or you can balance with the hands. Then seal the energy with CKR. Sealing means draw CKR in the aura. First draw a CKR from crown chakra to root chakra the draw another CKR from root chakra to the end of the body. Give little energy in aura also. Feel that patient received a good healing and will benefit from it. Pray the energy to continue the rapport till the next session. Chant the prayers. Now the session is closed.

You can scan the body if needed; scan can be done in the beginning of the session to know where energy is needed. If it is done after the session then it is done to know did all parts received energies or not. Slowly call the patient if he is slept. If he is in a deep sleep then stop calling after two or three times. Let him have rest for some more time.

Healing is more effective if the patient gets the maximum sleep. Sleeping means relaxation; only in this relaxation body will get the ability to heal. Wash your hands before and after the treatment. It is a good procedure to wash the hands with salt water after the treatment while treating chromic ailments.

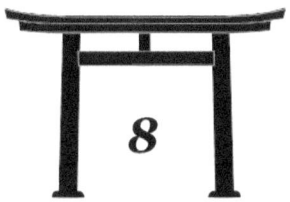

8   *Reiki Hand positions*

Reiki energy flows smoothly and effectively within the patient's body through the practitioner hand, hence a definite sequence hand positions are important. There may be variations in hand positions from teacher to teacher. The important thing is; when you place the hand in the body, energy will start to spread out where it is needed, regardless of your hand positions. Still, we should follow a particular hand positions in the preliminary stage, and in the advanced stage it can be altered. Whole body treatment can be given by leaving your hands in just one place; however by doing the hand placements, you assure that each area gets a surcharge of the Reiki, and all of the major meridian channels are treated. In advanced stages, Reiki is given to the positions, which are identified by sensations.

The basic set of hand positions is nearly eighteen for self-treatment and nearly twenty-two for healing others. These hand positions cover all the major energy channels, chakras and aura. It is assumed that, Usui used five basic hand placements only and treated further areas if needed. Dr Hayashi is the architect of hand positions we now use. These hand positions are also used in other traditional Japanese and Chinese healing modes thus not exclusive to Reiki.

Hand

Before administering any of these positions; hold both hands with palms down, facing the body of the patient. Extend and hold the fingers and thumb together, making an arch, so that a hollow is created under the palms. Splayed fingers or flat palms might allow the energy to dissipate. Do not let the recipient cross his/her legs or arms. Reiki touch is very light, so, no pressure is applied. The energies often run for about 3 to 5 minutes in each position.

Note: This healing methodology written below is from the Tantric knowledge; it is not yet proven by medical science. In my personnel experience; I have found that it has a rational basis, and got results in my healing sessions. I have also referred the book "Transform your life with Reiki by Anil Bhatnagar" while writing this section.

Head positions

The head positions; it is considered as the most important positions of the human body. You can evaluate the whole body, and character of the patient from the sensations of the head. You should give treatment to the four head positions to each and every type of diseases regardless whether disease is for head or not. It can be given either by, sitting or standing behind the patient's head. The patient can sit upright on a chair, or lie down on his or her back on a massage table or a mattress placed on the floor. The best way always is in lying down on the massage table.

Position 1: Eye

To treat yourself: Cup the eyes with your palms, with your fingers on the forehead and the sides of your palm comfortably placed on the sides of the nose. Let the smallest finger of each hand meet the third eye.

To treat others: Sit or stand behind the head and place your arched palms on the eyes. The thumbs of both hands should touch near the middle of the eyebrows. Place your fingers comfortably on the sides of the patient's nose, taking care not to hinder or constrict the nostrils.

Chakra involved: Third eye or Aagnya

Physical level: All strains and stress of the body is reflected in the eyes and the face in the body. When the eyes are relaxed the body is relaxed. Healing in this position relieves eye strain and arrests the deteriorating of the vision. It heals eye problems such as glaucoma, cataracts, detached retina etc., and problems relating to the pineal or pituitary glands. Other major diseases are Sinuses, colds, flu, allergies and coughs. Radiations from television and computers are reduced. It gives complete refreshment to the entire face which enables the eye-Sight, taste and smell to get more sensitive. It is an important point for brain tumors which originates from headaches. Treatment can be given up to 20 minutes.

Mental and emotional level: Mind enjoys peace and remains calm. Addictions and allergies initiates to melt down. Feel refreshed on the whole day.

Energy level: By healing here, we will get the maximum energy to work for whole day and will not feel drained. Enhanced intuition and clairvoyance is also obtained.

Position 2: Temples

To treat yourself: Place your palms on your temples (between your eyes and ears). Each palm should be somewhere between the eye and the earlobe.

To treat others: Place your palms on the temples, with the tips of your fingers reaching the cheek bones. Keep your fingers and the thumbs together.

Chakra: Crown or Sahasraram

Physical level: It is considered as an important spot in yoga. There is an outlet in the center of the head; through this outlet everything (oils etc) is reached inside the head. Through this outlet prana entered in the body and also departed (death) through it. So it can be considered as the center of the body. Healing in this position relaxes the eye muscles, local nerves and other muscles radiating out from the jaw. It heals colds, headaches, earaches and problems relating to the pineal or pituitary glands. All the disease (tumors, memory loss etc) regarding brain should be treated mainly on this region.

Mental and emotional level: It brings tranquility by healing depression, manic depression or general anxiety. All the passions such as anger, worries, melancholy, likes and dislikes, guiltiness and disgust can be minimized. It stimulates the brain and achieves its utmost potency. Concentration, creativity and Memory level is raised.

Energy level: it is the spot of happiness, so you will always feel happy and energetic. The capability to achieve lofty levels increases. Progress to the inner world fastens and obtains the gift of rational thinking. It is the gateway of prana, so, Reiki assist to depart this life serenely to those patients who are seriously ill. Patient's fear of the death and worry about the future of their relatives are peacefully solved.

Position 3: Ears

To treat yourself: Place your cupped palms on your ears.

To treat others: Same as above.

Chakra: Third eye or Aagnya

Physical level: It is considered as the life point. The sound (like burning of fire or wheels of the moving horse cart) inside the ear is considered as the existence of prana inside the body. This sound is heard only when a person is alive, so it is considered as the divine sound of prana. We will not perceive this sound when we are reaching the death. Hence the ears are important positions for any kind of ailment; it keeps our bodies in balance. Like the palms of the hand and soles of the feet, the ears are 'circuit boards' comprising nerve endings from most major parts of the body; they hold a number of important acupuncture points connecting the major energy meridians. Providing Reiki at this position can improve hearing loss, balance problems. There is also a connection between nasal and ears so colds can be healed. It is also an important point for fever and pressure variations. Sinus problems can also be healed in this region. Radiations from the mobile phones can be reduced while healing here.

Mental and emotional level: it boosts the intuitive power and the ability to solve the problems. It augments our listening power and hearing others view point. It increases the quality of mercy and magnanimity in life.

Energy level: mind and body accomplish balanced.

Position 4: Occipital Lobes

The occipital lobe is the rearmost lobe in each hemisphere of the brain.

To treat yourself: Cup the occipital lobes where the throat meets the lower back of the skull.

To treat others: Cradle the back of the head in your relaxed palms. The sides of the palms should touch, with the fingers reaching the base of the skull.

Chakra: Aagnya

Physical level: All the nerves and nadis are centered in this point. So it is considered as the most important part in the head positions. By healing this position whole part of the body is healed. It is an important point in reducing the anxieties, fear, pressure variations and pains which may have symptoms from head to leg. It relieves headaches and fevers, it also heals circulatory disorders and problems stemming from cerebellum and spinal fluid, the brain's visual cortex, the large intestine, the gall bladder and what Chinese medicine calls the governor vessel, thus promoting a sense of serenity and balance. It helps in healing asthma, headaches, colds, abdominal complaints, emphysema, pneumonia, hyperventilation, sneezing, nausea and insomnia and other sleep disorders.

Mental and emotional level: Heals anger, disappointment, anxiety and frustration. We can make best use of the creative and thinking aspects of the brain. Mind will always get a cooling effect rather than heated. It accomplishes balance and co-ordination between the hemisphere of the brain and between the pituitary and pineal glands. It regulates breathing, heartbeat, muscle movement and digestion.

Energy level: intellectual facility widens the horizons and we are able to perceive spiritual thoughts. It heals absent-mindedness.

Position 5: Throat

To treat yourself: Slide one hand under the hollow of the neck and bring the other over the throat. Keep the fingers and thumbs of both hands together.

To treat others: Same as above. Let the edge of the upper palm take support from the patient's collar bone so he or she does not feel pressure on the wind pipe. Alternately, the palms can be kept at sides of the throat.

Chakra: Vishudhi or Throat.

Physical level: Throat is the mother of all words and also the position in which our waking state remains. Healing in this position alleviates the vocal cords and specific speech problems such as hoarseness and stammering. It releases the breath and increases the flow of energy to whole body the thyroid gland regulates metabolism and balances blood pressure and cleanses the lymphatic system. All neck stiffness, auto immune diseases (not AIDS) and dental problems can be healed. It eases general stress. It heals clogged sinuses, weight problems, swollen glands, gum disease, throat and mouth ulcers, anorexia, osteoporosis, palpitation, poor posture, shoulder tension, problems in the pelvic region and legs, sore throat, laryngitis, tonsillitis and other throat ailments, and problems relating to the thyroid and parathyroid glands(for the assimilation of calcium and magnesium), and throat cancer.

Mental and emotional level: It allows you to present something comfortably. Inability of expressions and under- or over-expression vanishes. You will get control over the voice. Voice will become more melodious.

Energy level: Heals addictive behavioral patterns.

Position 6: Shoulders/ Lungs

To treat yourself: place your palms over your shoulders, at the sides of your neck. If you find this difficult, you may cross your arms so that each palm touches the opposite shoulder. Alternately, hold one palm over the opposite shoulder, near the neck, and place the other palm over the kidney on that side. Repeat on the other shoulder. If you adopt this variation, you may skip the kidney position.

To treat others: Place your palms over the shoulders, parallel to each other. Alternately, place your palms in a straight horizontal line across the shoulder blades, with the Fingertips of the hand closer to you touching the heel of the other palm.

Chakra involved: Throat

Physical level: Shoulders hold the responsibility of the whole body. If a person is mentally weak then it is reflected in the shoulders. Healing in this position improves the circulation of the arms and result in free movements of hand. Joints of the bones feel stronger. It helps in healing lung problems, particularly beneficial for smokers, people with asthma and people living in polluted cities. It liberates accumulated tension in the neck and shoulder regions. It heals headaches. It activates the parasympathetic nervous system (which calms the body when necessary) and, when combined with abdominal positions, improves digestion through the autonomic nervous system.

Mental and emotional level: It heals laziness and fear. Releases stress and heals responsibility issues, such as overestimating or failing to admit one's personal responsibilities. It helps the person to initiate relationship that he has avoided for fear or rejection.

Energy level: It helps you to be confident, take responsibilities and believe in your selves.

Torso positions

If you are giving Reiki to someone else, these positions will be easier if you stand on one side of the torso

Position 7: Heart

To treat yourself: keep your lower hand where it is but move the upper one below it, still adjacent.

To treat others: Same as above. However, when treating a woman, place one hand between the breasts and the other horizontally just above it (over the thymus gland), forming a T. If you are a male and not on intimate terms with your patient, keep your hands an inch or so above the breasts as a mark of respect for woman's privacy. You can also use this T variation for males if your intuition guides you to do so, or if you simply find yourself more comfortable with it. Alternately, place your left palm over your right palm above the heart. Though it is the heart chakra (placed right in the centre) and not the physical heart (which is slightly towards one's *l*eft), allow your hands to be guided a bit to one side by any pull or repulsion they experience.

Chakra: Heart or Anahatam

Physical level: It is the position where physical heart is located. Healing in this position alleviates cardiac problems, pneumonia, deafness, and lung cancer and auto immune disorders such as arthritis, chronic fatigue, general weakness, AIDS, cancer and TB etc. It enhances the vitality, makes stronger immune system and regulates the respiratory organs. It is an important point for asthma and hyper tension which directly affects the respiratory system.

Mental and emotional level: Rapport with mind amplifies. Able to perceive the inner voice undoubtedly, thereby attain solutions for your problems. It enhances feelings of trust and harmony. It heals emotional problems either lack of emotion or excess emotion.

Energy level: Intellect will peep into metaphysical effects or to the sources of physical heart. Magnanimity and compassion arouses from it.

Position 8: Solar plexus

To treat yourself: keep your hands above both sides of the navel.

To treat others: Same as above. Alternately, place the hands in a horizontal line across the solar plexus.

Chakra: Solar plexus or Manipurakam

Physical level: All tensions and karmic debts are stored in solar plexus, because it is the position of mind in the human body. If this position is healed then almost all the roots of diseases get healed. All the disease is due to unhealthy digestion. Undigested food later develops to serious illness. If your digestive organ is healthy then there will be no disease for you. It heals all the digestive organs (liver, stomach, gall bladder, spleen, alimentary canal) and thus helps healing digestive problems, gastric or duodenal ulcers, anorexia nervosa, bulimia, diabetes, colon and intestinal problems, arthritis, liver disorders, fat around the middle of the body, headaches and fevers.

Mental and emotional level: All passions such as tension, worry, anger and lust get healed here. The inability to take responsibility and make decisions and power-struggle issues improves. Fears, getting nervous in situation and anxiety for future problems are burned out.

Energy level: Improves self confidence and gains strength to face any challenges in adversity. It minimizes the worry of getting ill, hence always enjoys good health. Mind also gets more concentration if it is free from risks.

Position 9: Liver/Gall bladder/ Pancreas/Spleen

To treat yourself: Keep your hands on both sides of the navel.

To treat others: Same as above. Alternately, place the hands in a horizontal line across the spleen, across the depression where the lower ribs meet in front.

Chakra: Solar plexus or Manipurakam

Physical level: If liver is lost everything is lost, because liver is the filter of the body. All toxins in the body either physical or mental are stored here. Hence you should not give intensive healing to those regions for the first few sessions because; it will result in immediate healing crisis. Toxins in the body particularly stored in this area should melt down slowly. When toxins in the body are removed then it improves the overall health of the body. Reiki has the capability to heal the liver even though it has lost 50% of it. It heals liver problems (such as jaundice), gall bladder problems, high blood pressure, hormonal imbalances, cholesterol problems, allergies, hemorrhoids, headaches and metabolic diseases. It helps healing indigestion, diabetes, hypoglycemia, rheumatoid arthritis and all kind of infections.

Mental and emotional level: It heals fears, suppressed anger and other repressed aggressive emotions. It improves decision-making ability. It heals the tendency to manipulate and/or be manipulated, and an excess or dearth of sweetness

Energy level: Improves judgment. It enables us to achieve goals. It fine tunes the relationship between ideals and what one actually practices. Cultivates equanimity, tranquility, sweetness and meaningfulness

Position 10: Navel/Hara

To treat yourself: Place one hand above the navel and the other below it.

To treat others: Same as above.

Chakra: Hara or Swadhistanam

Physical level: This portion is the energy spot of survival and sexual activities; hence it is the spot of vitality. Sex is also considered as the mother of creativity. Healing in this position improves overall health. It heals all the problems related to sexual and reproductive organs. Drawing Reiki in this position, along with the root chakra, can even heal the problems of fertility for both individuals. It enhances the digestive process. It helps in

healing metabolic and gastrointestinal diseases, nausea, bloat-
ing, hemorrhoids, prostate and bladder disorders, cervical and
prostate cancer, fibroids, tumors, allergies, pelvic and lower
back pain, skin disorders, addictions and overindulgence in alcohol, sex or food.

Mental and emotional level: It heals emotional scars, depression and anxiety. It improves intuition and brings inner peace
and harmony. All suppressed feelings and unsolved problems in the unconscious mind reveals to the surface and will
be completely healed. (Men, because they tend to have more
suppressed feelings than women, tend to draw more Reiki in
this position). It boosts the ability to enjoy physical and sexual
pleasures.

Energy level: improves the stamina which triggers the quality
and pleasure of sex. It brings peace and stability. It will awake
the dormant creativity.

Position 11: Groin

To treat yourself: Form a V with your palms over the pelvic
bones, and adjust until your hands cover the genitals. Keep
your fingers and thumbs together.

To treat others: Same as above, but it might be more convenient to point the forehand in the opposite direction (i.e., point
the closer hand towards the things and the farther hand away
from them). Preserve your patient's privacy by keeping your
hand just above his or her body.

Chakra involved: Root or Mooladharam

Physical level: It is the seat of kundalini in which infinite energy is accumulated. It is the connection point between matter
and energy. Healing this chakra can eradicate as well as attain almost anything. Generally it heals physical and emotional

problems relating to the urinary and reproductive systems. It improves appetite, immunity, circulation and digestion. It may prevent the development of ovarian cysts and breast tumors in women and prostate problems in men. It also heals allergies, weight problems, migraine headaches, Menopause problems and general weakness, Aids in convalescence, Urogenital, digestive problems, chronic lower-back pain, sciatica and varicose veins. It can help in treating fissures, rectal tumors and cancers.

Mental and emotional level: Along with Occipital Lobes, spleen and knee; this is the vital point in healing all type of fears particularly fears from death. Our confidence level is raised to its maximum to face any adversity. It enhances the capability to broaden your horizon in the various fields of occult science and spiritual science. It cultivates good qualities such as magnanimity, simplicity, humbleness and obedience. It resolves sexual issues, including fear of physical intimacy, low sex drive, fear of intimacy, aversion to sexual intercourse, sexual perversion and sexual addiction. It heals lack of will to live or to enjoy life.

Energy level: Never feel drained. Makes one feel grounded and centered.

Position 12: Kidneys/adrenal glands

To treat yourself: Place your palms in a horizontal line across your back, one palm width above the waist (in line with the lower ribs), fingertips touching.

To treat others: Same as above, but you may find it more convenient to point the fingertips of the far hand away from you (touch the fingertips of one hand to the heel of the other palm).

Chakra: Swadhistanam.

Physical level: This portion is the filtering portion of the body. Healing in this position reduces kidney problems and helps prevent kidney failure in case of serious shock. It releases toxins stored in kidneys. It can heal sexual problems, infertility, allergies, and acrophobia. It maintains digestive organs and sympathetic nerve balance. Regular healing in this area prolongs life and preserves youthfulness.

Mental and emotional level: Filters out ideas and concepts that have outgrown their utility. It relieves stress. It Helps to heal partnership or relationship problems. It heals the fear of intimacy.

Energy level: It heals relationships and also a change the interpretation of relationship.

Leg positions

You can either treat two knees jointly or separately. If you are doing it separately then hold one hand above the knee and other hand under the knee.

Position 13: Knees

To treat yourself: Assume a sitting posture and cup your knees with your hands.

To treat others: Same as above. Alternately, treat each knee separately by placing both hands on one knee at a time—one above and the other at the back, in the hollow of the Joint. This variation is preferable for those with stiff or weak knee joints, those under stress, those confronting and fearing a particular change in life or those who generally
Find it emotionally difficult to face life's challenges with courage.

Chakra: Minor chakras in the knee region.

Physical level: Healing in this position relieves arthritic knees and all other sever knee problems like ortho-arthsis and rheumato-arthsis.

Mental and emotional level: It is a major point in healing anxiety and fear particularly related with future aspect. It helps to dissolve stubbornness, arrogance, fear of death or any unyielding attitude that keeps us from letting go, moving ahead and facing change.

Energy level: it dissolves excessive fears and attachments relating to insecurity, uncertainty and prospects for change. It enhances humility, empathy, tolerance and forgiveness.

Position 14: Left Foot

To treat yourself: Hold your left foot with both hands in a way that is comfortable.

To treat others: hold the left foot with both hands in a way that is comfortable to you.

Chakra involved: Muladharam.

Physical level: This area covers all 32 meridian points or reflex points. Feet's are equal to head. All the major points can be covered by healing the feet (It is also similar with the hands particularly the right hand). It is important to activate all the meridian point, hence walking with bare foot for 30 minutes is a must. All the parts such as solar plexus, sciatic nerves, gall bladder, ureters, small intestine, transverse and ascending colon, duodenum, pancreas, kidneys, stomach, lungs, gonads, and knees will get healing. Digestive system, the pelvic joint and muscles, the ovaries or testes and the lymphatic system are also other major points. Dissolves blocks in the flow of energy from the feet to the Muladharam. It can help in relieving those patients who are recovering from coma, anesthesia or any kind of shock.

Mental and emotional level: It gives relaxation to mind and body.

Energy level: It dissolves almost all energy blocks

Position 15: Left Toes

You can either treat both toes separately or jointly. If you are doing it joints then place your hands on both toes.

To treat yourself: Hold your left toe with both hands in a way that is comfortable.

To treat others: Hold your left toe with both hands in a way that is comfortable.

Chakra: Muladharam

Physical level: For heart problems and diabetic problems toes can be considered as one of the major important point. It also strengthens the Muladharam.

Mental and emotional level: it grounds all the chakras—that is, stabilizes their spin by connecting them to the center of Mother Earth through a thin, laser-like column of energy. One feels grounded when healed.

Energy level: Increase energy flow in nerve/naadi systems.

Positions 16-17: Right Foot and Toes

Repeat positions 16-18 on the left foot. There is no major difference between left and right food in healing.

Back positions

The back represents support, both financial (lower back) and emotional (upper back). Optional one, it is mainly used to treat others; if the client has back problems, asthma, and lung problems. If your intuition indicates to treat back then heal it. The back often receives Reiki when treating front parts of the body.

Position 18: Back of thyroid

It is an optional position for throat. You can skip this if you had treated in the front position of neck (position: 5 mentioned above and results much same)

To treat yourself: Bring your palms together at the back of your neck, one on top of the other.

To treat others: Have the patient lie on his or her stomach, head towards you. Place your palms together, one on top of the other, on the little protrusion at the base of the neck.

Chakra: Back of thyroid.

Position 19: Back of heart

To treat yourself: Bring your palms back from their respective sides and thrust them up towards the heart level as far they can go. Upturn them, letting the backs of the palms touch the body. Alternately, bring one hand from the top over the correspond-ing shoulder and the other up from below, to meet behind the heart. Both palms should face the body.

To treat others: Place your palms in a straight horizontal line across the shoulder blades, with the fingertips of one hand touching the heel of the other palm.

Chakra: Back of heart.

Physical level: It is the important point in healing asthma and other lung diseases. If patient is suffering from asthma first treat this position for at least 15 minutes. Heart problems are also benefited while treating here.

Mental and emotional level: Manic depressions and other emotional problems get relaxed.

Energy level: Breathing gets more regulated which enhance an energetic feeling through out the day.

Position 20: Back of hara

To treat yourself: Same as Position 10 but one palm width below, just above the buttocks. Results are same as 10.

To treat others: Same as above but touch the fingertips of one hand to the heel of the other palm.

Chakra involved: Back of hara.

Position 21: Muladharam

Result much the same as postion-11

To treat yourself: Place both hands on the tailbone, with the right one touching the tailbone and the left one above it. Alternately, bring your right hand form the front beneath the coccyx (the bottom-most triangular bone at the base of the spinal column) and the left hand from the back to cover the perineum (the area between the anus and the genitals).

To treat others: Place one hand over and along the fold of the buttocks and the other perpendicular to it, forming a T.

Chakra: Muladharam.

Diseases to treat via chakras

Disease	Chakras & Organs
Abortion	Anahatam, Manipurakam, Swadhistanam and Muladharam
Arthritis	All chakras
Astma	Anahatam, Manipurakam and Lungs in front and back
Back pain	At the spot and the near Chakra.
Bad habits	All Chakras
Breathing strain	Vishudhi, Anahatam and lungs.
Burning	Manipurakam Anahatam Muladharam Liver and Lungs
Cancer & Aids	Whole body
Cold	Vishudhi, Anahatam, head and Shoulders
Constipation	Muladharam Swadhistanam Manipurakam and Liver
Cough and sneezing	Vishudhi, Manipurakam and Lungs.
Cuts, wounds	Manipurakam Anahatam Muladharam Liver, Lungs and Places of wounds

Depression & Suicide tendency	Whole body
Diabetics	Manipurakam, Muladharam, Liver, Pancreas and hand joins
Fever	Manipurakam, Muladharam, Liver and Head
Headache	Manipurakam, Head, Neck and Feet
Heart attack	Anahatam Manipurakam and Muladharam
High BP	Swadhistanam, Kidney point and Knees
Indigestion	Manipurakam, Swadhistanam and Liver
Itching	Anahatam, Manipurakam and itching area
Jaundice	Manipurakam Liver and Kidney
Joint pain	Place of the pain and the nearest Chakras
Lack appetite	Manipurakam, Swadhistanam, Muladharam and place one hand in the front and other at the back of the Stomach for at least 20 minutes

Loose Motion	Manipurakam, Swadhistanam, Muladharam
Low BP	Muladharam, Anahatam and Knee
Lunacy	Sahasraram, Manipurakam Anahatam Muladharam
Piles	Muladharam, Swadhistanam
Pimples	Swadhistanam, Muladharam, liver and face
Prostrates problems	Swadhistanam Muladharam and feet
Skin disease	Muladharam and Liver, Places of disease
Sleeplessness	Anahatam, Manipurakam, Kidney and Head
Stomach pain	Manipurakam, Swadhistanam and Liver
Tension	Muladharam Swadhistanam, Knee and Head positions
Tonsillitis	Vishudhi, Anahatam, Muladharam and Manipurakam
Venereal diseases	Swadhistanam, Muladharam, Anahatam, Vishudhi and private parts
Vomiting sensations	Manipurakam Anahatam Swadhistanam and Aagnya

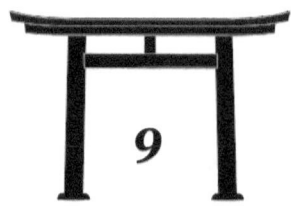

9   *Reiki Practitioner*

Legal aspects

When you become a Reiki practitioner, it is important to be aware of these legal aspects when working with people. You cannot legally Heal or Cure, diagnose, or prescribe. Only a medical doctor can do these things. You may get in trouble for practicing medicine without a license. Avoid these words - cure-diagnose-prescribe so as to avoid legal risk. There is another reason we do not use these words we in fact do not heal. WE allow the universal energy (Reiki) to flow through us and the universal energy is healing not us. The energy knows what to do; it comes from the INTENT to heal. Do not be attached to results, as you cannot make a mistake in the application of the energy. On a physical level when you touch you are healing. When someone comes to you it is he or she who needs you expertise, thus it cannot be considered as an illegal activity in medical field.

Professional Ethics of the healer

1. Healers should conduct themselves in a professional and ethical manner, perform only those services for which they are qualified and represent their education, certification, professional affiliations and other qualifications honestly.

2. He should present Reiki in a professional and compassionate manner, representing themselves and their practice accurately and ethically. Their practice should be honest, and should not give fraudulent information, nor misrepresent themselves to

students or clients, nor act in a manner derogatory to the nature and positive intentions of Reiki.

3. He/she should keep accurate client records, including profiles of the body, mind, and health history.

4. Before healing, he has to make sure the disease is properly diagnosed by the medical practitioner otherwise it will create unnecessary disputes among the medical fraternity.

5. Never play with patient's life. He should refer to the doctor, those cases in which he is not sure of or has questions about. It is better to treat patients when they have tried and failed with all other modalities. Reiki is new to our society and some people cannot digest the healing ability of Reiki so it is good to get the medical advice. These things are sometimes done just to satisfy a patient's relative.

6. They should pay close attention to cleanliness and professional appearance of self and clothing, and keep a professionally maintained clinic. They should endeavor to provide a relaxing atmosphere, furnish details about the working of Reiki, the healing crisis, sessions required to heal, and clarity about fees.

7. They should maintain clear and honest communication with their clients, and keep all client information, whether medical or personal, strictly confidential.

8. Establish and maintain a trustful relationship with the patient as they are encouraged to ask caring questions about the client's well-being, and to establish boundaries for a peaceful atmosphere for wellbeing.

9. They should respect the client's physical/emotional state, and not abuse clients through actions, words or silence, nor take advantage of the therapeutic relationship.

10. They should consider the client's comfort zones to touch and amount of pressure applied to the body and honor the client's requests as much as possible within personal, professional and ethical limits.

11. He/she should refrain from abuse of alcohol and drugs. These substances should not be used at all during professional activities.

12. He should possess the quality of learning. Never think that you have studied all. Assess your strengths and weaknesses, and overcome it by education and training. All the truth and wisdom lies within you. All you need to do is to develop your ability to listen. Listen from the inner mind. Learn from   observation. Learn from experience.

13. We should treat all channels and masters as equals without regard to their lineage or their belief.

Setting up a Treatment Room

A treatment room is not required to do Reiki; all that is necessary is placing your hands on the body (yours or the recipient's); sitting, standing or lying down. Still a good atmosphere is required for better healing. Ensure there are no unnecessary noises e.g. doors squeaking, curtains flapping, clocks ticking. If possible have the room at a comfortable temperature, avoid noisy heaters or fans if possible. Have a jug of fresh water and glasses near by for thirst. Before commencing Reiki when there is more than one giver discuss your procedures prior to commencement to avoid added distractions during the Reiki. As Reiki is an exchange of Universal Energy between a giver/and receiver, respect the solemnness of the occasion and ensure that all possible steps are taken, allow all persons to respect this energy. If you choose to set up a treatment room here are some guidelines:

- Select a room away from high traffic areas.
- Create a safe, relaxing, quiet atmosphere. Use soft colors, blinds over windows, plants, etc.
- Dim the lights or light candles to help the client relax.
- Ensure that the room is clean and tidy
- Ensure that there is good ventilation
- Ensure that the room is pleasant to the senses e.g.; burn incense or oils

Here are some additional guidelines:

- Place the massage table in the room so it is possible to move completely around it.
- A shelf, table or bookcase is a good place to put a CD/tape player, tissues, blanket and any other items you wish to include in your room.
- Aromatherapy diffuser and oils or add pleasant aromas which is an aid for relaxation.
- Place a fresh flower/s in the room to introduce nature

Equipment Needed:

A massage table, comfortable rolling chair, pillows (for head and under knees), tissue and blankets, CD/tape player, collection of soft soothing music. Provide suitable music to calm the mind, to place you or the recipient in a relaxed state. If a telephone is near, switch off to avoid unnecessary distractions.

Keeping a Reiki Journal

Keeping record is always good. We can understand the results of the healing. We can also show this to other person as a proof of our healing. In today world it is important to keep a good record because the false results are more than real results. Hence a healing forum will clear the doubts of the third party. It will be a proof if any disputes arise. Here is an example of healing form.

Sample Patient Information Form

(Signed by the patient or relative)

I have understood that Reiki practitioners neither diagnose conditions nor they prescribe substances, they neither perform medical treatment nor do they interfere with the treatment of a licensed medical professional in other modalities. They have recommended me to see a licensed physician, or licensed health care professional for any complicated ailment I may have. I should recognize that a Reiki treatment program must be followed to be truly effective, just like prescribed medication is only effective if taken as directed. I understand Reiki is a relaxation and rejuvenation therapy that also provides healing. Every system has their own science for healing and concepts about diseases, which may or may not be similar to other treatment modalities concepts. I should also understand and believe that the body has the ability to heal itself, to do so complete relaxation is often beneficial. Long-term imbalances in the body sometimes require multiple treatments to allow the body to reach the level of relaxation necessary to bring the system back into balance. I should understand and believe that self-improvement requires commitment on my part, and I must be willing to change in a positive way if I have to receive the full benefit of Reiki treatment. I am also acknowledging Reiki Practitioner's commitment to my self-improvement process whole heartedly.

Signed: _____

Print Name: _____

Date: _____

Address: _____

City: _____

State: _____ Zip: _____

Phone: _____

List treatments or medications client is currently receiving? Medication or Treatment Type Dosage or Frequency When did they start

Comments and history

Reiki Treatment Documentation Form
Patient Name: _____
Date: _____
Treatment start time: _____
End time: _____

Treatment notes:

Indicate the reason client has come to you and the areas where blockages and/or Releases were felt. Identify blockages in the appropriate energy body, Physical, Emotional or Mental. Has there been any change in client condition, medications or dosages, (recommended by doctor) other treatment programs, or environment, etc. that should be noted?

Practitioner Signature: _____

Date: _____

Additional treatment notes or drawings:

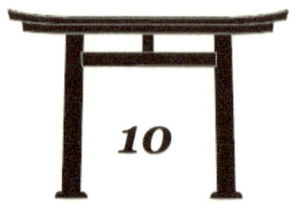

10   *Distant & Group Healing*

"Enkaku Chiryo ho" is the Japanese name for Distant Reiki or Absentee Reiki treatment. One specific distant technique Usui taught was called "Shashin Chiryo ho" or Photograph healing. This practice used a photograph of the person as a focus or "proxy" for healing. While having a photograph is nice, anything can be used as a proxy or representation of the person. There are so many methods in distant healing. Object can be anything, which has less important, and the Visualization has the prime importance while treating.

- Visualizing treating the patient from your place
- Visualizing treating the patient in the patient place
- Visualizing the patient is become too small and encircled in the hand.
- Visualizing the patient's body in a pillow
- Visualizing the patient in a photo.

Choose any one among them, which you feel convenient. Chant the prayer of Reiki. Draw all the three symbols in the order and chant their names respectively. Ask the permission from the patient to whom you are giving Reiki. Patient has the choice of accepting or rejecting it. Say thanks to the vital energy and let the patient may accept or may not accept this healing and you are ready to start the healing proceedings. After that, draw the HSZSN and imagine that you are creating a bridge between yourself and the patient with the HSZSN.

After that, hold the hands in a blessing position and imagine that you are giving Reiki to the patient. If you are giving it to objects such as pillow or photo, touch your hands on the object and visualize it as a body.

You can choose one from the either methods, Change the hand positions just like in a whole body treatment or not identifying the body as different part but as a whole body. Give it till you feel satisfied because there is no time limit for distant healing. At most times you will get the sensation that patient is taking the energy, after a while sensation starts to diminish and eventually stops, which means that energy is full and he received the healing. This is distant healing. The energy here acts as a bridge between space and time or past, present and future. Distance among healer and patient is makes no difference and healing is also much same as treating with touch.

There are some conditions to give distant. Among them the main one is patient should not be in a distance in which we can reach quickly. Never do distant if you can heal him directly or he is nearby from you. There should be genuine distance between them. You cannot give distant while patient is in the next house or nearby. There should also be a genuine reason for giving distant. .Give distant healing only on emergency situations. Distant healing is considered as an ultimate weapon just like atom bomb so use it cautiously. Do not take it as a child's play. Reiki is not a tool used in a childish way rather it should be given seriously.

Childish does not mean that a child cannot receive attunements. Children's are more serious and sincere than professional healers. This determination or lack of seriousness and sincerity is termed as childish. Secondly the patient is genuinely needed healing. Thirdly patient should request distant. It should never be the choice of the healer to give distant but from the choice of patient or his relatives. Reiki should be given only by the request whether it is distant or laying hands in the physical body. Distant can be given from the choice of the healer in those cases where the patient is in an unconscious state or in ICU. In all the other cases it should be from the choice of the patient or his relatives.

The usual procedure of distant healing is as follows. First the patient or relatives who want the distant should make the request and healer agrees it. After that, fix a convenient time to suit the both persons. Tell that time to the patient and ask him to lie comfortably at that time either in bed or chair. He should avoid walking or any similar activities during that time like watching TV or computers.

Patient should be in a relaxed mood during that time that is why requesting him to lie down. Let his mind may be disturbed or relaxed but his body should be relaxed. After the healing patient or the relatives should inform the healer what they felt or about the present condition after the distant. If they want distant in the next days then they should make the request for that. The procedures should be the similar above. Get feed back every day. If they are not giving any feedback discontinue the distant healing. It is better to give distant for seven days continuously and stop after it, but in some cases we have to continue for some more time.

Group Healing

Group Healing or Shuchu Reiki is taught as the traditional method of a Reiki Group Treatment. This technique was taught by Usui, Hayashi and Mrs. Takata. Group healing sessions are an especially powerful experience not only for the person being worked on, but also for the practitioners involved. Group healing is done mainly for chronic patient particularly who is near to death. It is also done to less the burden with practitioners. More and more person's added will also reduces the treatment time. Group healing increases the healing much faster than normal healing.

It is a technique, which concentrates Reiki energy more than one-person. The energy is intensified with each additional practitioner that joins the treatment. Several practitioners form a group and heal on one patient. One person will treat one spot and the other at a different spot. For example one treats head other in the stomach etc. Hand potions are moved according to it. It is not needed to treat a spot where other person has already healed. It is also good if one person give aura healing while other give touch healing. It is a collective effort than a single effort. It is much more powerful than a single treatment. All the parts of the body are getting energized in the same time is the highlights of this treatment. Patient will get the maximum healing so he is benefited more with it. If two persons have joined as a group in healing then it is equal to two individual sessions. If three persons have joined as a group in healing then it is equal to three individual sessions. Similarly it will pile up with the adding of healers. It is important that in-group treatment the channels which join together should have the same wave length in thoughts and deeds. The outlook of them should not be different. If it is different then it will create tensions.

*Different types of group healing**

There are many ways to conduct such sessions, depending on how many practitioners are present, and what their level of training is. Experiment yourself and see what works for you, develop your own methods, and you will be well on your way to becoming an exceptionally powerful healer.

1. Reiki Mawashi - The traditional method of Reiki Circle

A group of Reiki practitioners make a circle holding hands. Then let the Reiki flow from one hand to the other, resulting in the strong flow of energy in people's circle. We do this with a slight variation. In this technique two or more practitioners join together and start to beam in the aura of a patient. The word Mawashi means 'round, game, revolve, current'.

In Dr. Hayashi's clinic in Japan, the practitioners worked in teams. Group sessions involve several Reiki practitioners working on one client all at the same time. This has the benefit of allowing many people to be treated more rapidly. It is also a blissful and pleasant experience. Groups generally consist of 2 to 4 practitioners. (Any more than that and it gets crowded!!!). To organize a group, designate someone the leader, that person does the head positions. Divide up evenly the remaining positions with the other practitioners. Have people change positions at the same time as instructed by the leader. This way everyone starts and finishes about the same time.

2. The traditional method

If the group consists solely of first level practitioners, there are several ways of conducting the session. The first is to have each person place their hands in one of the suggested healing positions. If there are not enough practitioners to fill every position, simply rotate after an appropriate amount of time. Many prefer to rotate even when there are more than enough healers present. This gives everyone the chance to experience the energy in different parts of the client's body, and thus gain additional experience.

When there is an excess of practitioners, allow the additional ones to take up positions at other areas of the body such as the ankles, shoulders, and knees in that order. These areas serve as bridges linking the energy in the two sides of the client's body together into a sort of grand circuit. The ankles usually do the best job of completing that link. Many say the knees are places where resistance to change is held in the body. Keep in mind that when placing your hands on them, if there is no one at the ankles, it will form a bridge of energy at the knees largely ignoring the rest of the legs.

If there is only one additional practitioner, it is usually best if they begin at the ankles and spend some time there before moving up to the knees. The shoulders are also an excellent place to use in balancing out the energy polarity in the body. After placing one hand on each shoulder, you should be able to feel the energy more strongly in one at first and later feel them balance out. This is an especially nice thing to experience when you are first beginning to use Reiki.

3. Mirroring

A second way to conduct a group healing is to use a technique called mirroring. In this practice, instead of each healer having one hand position that they are responsible for, they share two positions with another practitioner. For instance, instead of just placing your hands over the solar plexus, you would place one hand over the solar plexus and the other hand on another area of the person's body, such as the second chakra.

The person directly across from you would then do the same, matching their hands up to yours. In this way, your hands are "mirroring" each other. This can be a very powerful technique as it ties together not only two peoples' energy, but also two areas of the client's body between them. As with everything else, experiment with both practices and choose the one, which you feel most comfortable with.

4. Group healing with first and second level practitioners

If one or more second level practitioners comprise the group, have one of them trace the symbols over the client before the healing begins. If there is only one-second level practitioner, that person usually takes up position at the head. The crown chakra position is the one, which calls in most of the energy during a session, and fills the client's field with energy. By having a second degree or higher practitioner at this position, a much broader spectrum of energy enters the client's field for the other practitioners to utilize.

If the person being worked on has a specific area of the body, which is giving them trouble, it may be more beneficial for the second degree practitioner to take a position in that area. As always, use your intuition. It is perfectly acceptable for practitioners of different degrees to mirror one another, or for some of the group to mirror, while others concentrate on a single position each. The only positions that are not conducive to mirroring are the head, legs (including the knees), feet and ankles. It is also best if the shoulders are not mirrored unless the goal is physical healing of that area, rather than balancing of the two sides of the client's body.

5. *The circle method*

The circle method is another fun technique to experiment with. It has a number of different applications and variations. The first one, which will cover, is the closed circle method. This is a quick and easy way for a group of Reiki practitioners to work on each other. Basically, it involves forming a circle with each practitioner facing the back of the person in front of them. Once you are in this position, there are several different ways to proceed.

My favorites include, placing your hands on the shoulder blades of the person in front of you, placing your hands on the back of the heart center of the person in front of you, or holding your hands one to six inches off the back of the person in front of you and beaming energy to them. Any of these works well, and there are many other versions of this listed in various books as well as in newsletters and handouts from various masters, which also work nicely.

There is not a set time attributed to this exercise, so simply continue to send the energy for as long as everyone wants to. One of the nice things about this technique is that not everyone in the circle has to be a Reiki practitioner. This is an ideal introductory tool to use, as non-Reiki people can take part in this powerful healing technique and still strongly feel the energy pass through them. If possible, stagger the non-Reiki people between practitioners attuned to second degree or higher.

This technique can also be utilized to send healing at a distance. There are, in fact, many different ways to do this. The simplest is for all second degree practitioners present to use a witness of some kind to represent the person (see the chapters on mental/emotional healing and distant healing for a further definition of this), trace the symbols over it in the manner you use for healing at a distance, and then hold it between their hands and the back of the person in front of them. The benefits of this method are two fold. First, the circle is not broken, and everyone participating in the healing session still receives full benefit from it. Second, the people or things being sent energy receive not only the energy you would normally be able to send, but the energy of everyone in the group as well. This makes it much more powerful than a normal distant healing.

If you prefer, you con use a broken circle to send group healing in this manner. To do this, simply decide who will be sending the energy, give this person the witnesses to send energy to, and have him or her create a distant healing stack out of them. Then, create a healing circle leading up to the person who has been elected to send the energy. This person, instead of holding his or her hands to the back of the next person, sends the energy only into the distant healing stack. Though this method is perfectly fine to use, I suggest using closed circle because of the added advantage of everyone in the group receiving additional healing as well.

6. *Group projecting*

This is an excellent way to begin a group healing session as it is done from outside most levels of the client's energy field, and subsequently many levels are treated at once. To utilize this method, simply form a circle around the person to be healed. Ten feet away is ideal, but any shorter distance will do. Hold your hands out in front of you, facing the client, and send energy in one of the ways listed in the chapter on treating without touching, under projecting energy. The distance method can be used here as well.

*Note – Taken from various Internet sources

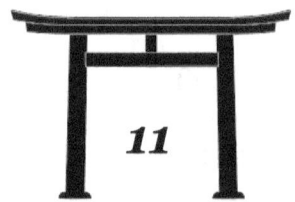

11   *Techniques*

Short description of scanning, beaming and sweeping are mentioned in the chapter healing session too.

1. Scanning

The roots of this method, as well as the projecting method of treatment, are found in the healing traditions of many cultures worldwide. Huna, Chinese energy medicine, traditional magic, and the increasingly common Therapeutic Touch type techniques all contain a wealth of information about this method.

This is done to find the stale energy in the aura and as well as in the body. This is not a diagnosing technique but we can feel the need of energy on those spots. These spots are often places of blocked energy or manifested illness and are usually among the first areas treated in a "hands-off" healing. Removal of these blocks will often increase the client's ability to draw energy and integrate it during the session so that later the energy can be focused in other places where it is needed. Never reveal those spots to the patient because it may fear the patient. Keep it in your mind and heal the area.

You can scan the body using your hands held about approximately 1-6 inches above the body. Move your hands slowly and systematically from the top of the head to the soles of the feet. Be aware of the sensations in your hand and when they detect anything different or feel a distortion in the energy field, your have found a place that needs Reiki. You may also feel this as tingling, pressure, and little electric shocks. Your hand maybe guided to the correct spot. As you practice your ability to scan the aura will improve. Finish scanning the entire body. Then give treatment to the distorted area. You can treat the patient in two ways.

At the end of the scanning by remembering the locations of stale energy.

When the time you found any irregularity in the person's energy field is a sign that you want to stop scanning for a moment and work on that area.

2. The Aura sweep

It is done to balance patient's energy field as well as in cleansing the surface of their aura of negative energy. This technique is mainly used in Pranic healing.

Lay the patient in the healing bed. Now, sweep your hands from above the top of their head, to the ground beneath them, and back several times. Do this by stretching your arms out in front of you with your fingers together and pointing at the person you are working on. As you sweep them from head to toe, visualize beams of energy coming from the tips of your fingers and passing through the person, removing all negative energy as they do so.

When you are done, shake your hands, as if you are shaking water from them, and ground the energy by cleansing yourself in one of the ways mentioned in the chapter on conducting a session. The easiest ways to ground yourself are washing your hands off in cold water, pressing them together in a Gassho for a minute or so, or placing them directly on the earth for thirty seconds to a minute.

3. Beaming

It is done at the end of the session. Healing the patient without touching his body or aura healing is known as beaming. We do beaming while healing distant.

There is no need to draw symbol if we are doing along (end or beginning) with treatment. If we are treating alone, visualize the symbols on your third eye or draw them in the air, chanting their names to yourself. Feel connected. Hold both hands at chest height, palms facing outward from you. Then simply send Reiki. You will feel it pour through your hands. As you send they will be receiving Reiki healing.

Other Healing Techniques*

It is said that energy emanates most strongly from the hands and this is why touch healing (Te-ate) is taught first in Reiki. Energy also emanates strongly from the eyes and the breath. So only the medium is changed and rest all are the same. The medium of hand is changed into breath or eyes. It is said that all Reiki is Karuna (compassionate action) and Metta (loving kindness). The essence of your being is loving-kindness for all.

There are number of ways to give Reiki. It can be either with hands or without hands. Even with hands there are again different methods. Follow any one of these methods or any method, which you feel, is comfortable. According to our observation after having a good healing experience each person will get a unique method, which suits him. Following that method is the best for you. That method may differ from all these method. We use a very different method in which all these seven qualities included. We have not forcefully created it but it came as bestow in intuition on our sessions. The stroking method is a powerful method it will get other method benefit along with Reiki. It activates all the meridian points and also gets the same result of massage. Blowing and sweeping is used in India even before Reiki originated. Our grand mothers and mothers used this technique to remove the negative energy from the body particularly caught by eyes.

In the interview already published in Reiki, The Legacy of Dr. Usui, Dr. Usui responded to the question of whether the Usui Reiki Ryoho uses medications and there would be any type of side effects: "It uses neither medications nor instruments. It uses only looking, blowing, stroking, (light) tapping and touching (of the afflicted part of the body). This is what heals diseases." Without these techniques, it would not be possible to understand the intuitive bodywork of Dr. Usui. The seven methods are:

1. Touching
2. Pushing/Pulsing
3. Tapping
4. Stroking
5. Blowing
6. Gazing
7. Specifically giving energy with one hand and raising the other hand.

1. Touching

This is the traditional healing method. Just place the hand in the body and move the hand to the next position after healing. This is the common method mainly followed in Reiki treatments.

Note: The next three are different in hand movements only. One is a light touch and one is hard and other is soft. The three techniques can be found in many Qi Gong books. All the three are just like a slow massage. The aims of theirs are: a slow massage can activate the meridian points and also increases the blood flow.

Blood flow and energy is blocked in these meridian points in a disease so by pressuring it the blockages are removed. The major difference between a massage and Reiki healer is; Reiki healer is pressuring the meridian points by applying Reiki energy. So it can augment the quality of both the massage as well as the Reiki.

2. Pushing /Pulsing.

Place the hand over the diseased area. Then open and close the palm very often so that energy passes through the center of the hand. The energy emerged from it enters the body very fast and heals it. Refection of the hand should be done in a rigid way. The indications for pulsing are similar to tapping. It stimulates and improves circulation. Pulsing can be used over any area of the body that requires it, including specific meridian points. If you pulse directly over a meridian point, it is easy to feel tingling and warmth at the point or radiating along the meridian.

3. Tapping

This means to lightly and rhythmically tap or pat the qi field with either your palm or fingertips. This technique is common to many forms of Chi Kung (qi- gong) and is used to help increase energy flow. This is useful to relieve stagnation or congestion and to improve circulation. In Tui-na Chinese Massage, tapping is applied directly to the body for the same purpose.

The intention of this technique is not to massage the area, rather to stimulate the body and allow the Reiki energy to penetrate into the body. The force used in patting is light to medium and it should not be a hard stuff. The therapist taps with either finger, palm, back of hand, side of hand, or fist to produce varying degrees of stimulation.

4. Stroking hand/Waving.

Is very useful for congestion or pain and also encourages the energy flow in the body. This technique is the fingertips sweep down the entire body. The hands are placed flat on the body in a circular way which enables to penetrate energy deep into skin. This is a quiet useful technique for alleviating pains. Only soft touch is required.

5. Blowing

It is the way of healing with the breath. This technique does not seem to have directly survived in Takata Sensei's teachings. It indirectly appears in many attunements where the Reiki Master "blows" the energy or symbols into the student. This technique is useful especially when you want to give Reiki to where you cannot touch, burned area or accident victim for an example. It is also useful for those who do not want touch treatment.

This is a focused way of healing with the breath. After connecting to Reiki, do Pranayama, which let your mind relaxed before giving Reiki treatment. Visualize the three symbols on the lips of your mouth. Inhale in through the nose. Exhale through the mouth. You are inhaling the vital energy and exhaling the same vital energy for healing. While exhaling assumes that, all symbols are there in the mouth. The lips form a small gate opening that the breath flows through it as a pass way and the energy is passing through this gate to the affected area. When the energy travels to the affected area imagine that all the three symbols are also traveling with it and reaching the affected area and finally merged to the affected area. Exhale the area till you feel it is healed.

6. Gazing

It is the way of healing with the Eyes. This technique is very useful to treat people that cannot be touched such as a burn, accident or abuse victim. In this technique we transfer the vital energy with the eyes. A compassionate look to the affected area's to be healed and feel that the area be cleansed and healed. Eyes are the reflections of your mind. All passions are reflected in it.

There are lots of examples from the divine personalities that, a compassionate look can change the character of a man or even make wild animals as a pet. Hence compassionate look itself has tremendous power when it merges with the healing they will radiate a powerful beam of healing.

Do not try hard to focus or glare on it. The look is not a "stare", but a soft, relaxed, defocused look. Just a compassionate look then we can see that the vital energy is radiating out from the eyes and traveling to the affected area. Like all other techniques this is also simple hence do it in a relaxed state.

After connecting to Reiki, when your eyes are relaxed then close your eyes and visualize the three symbols in the eyes. While looking think that, all symbols are there in the eyes. Symbols are the gates. Energy flows through the symbols to the affected area. Imagine the energy radiating from the eyes like the powerful beams of light. When the rays are traveling to the affected area imagine that all the three symbols are also traveling with it and reaching the affected area and finally merged to the affected area or the rays of light is burning the affected area. Look the area till you feel it is healed.

7. Healing through one hand

One Japanese Reiki School teaches that Dr. Usui received the Reiki energy with his left hand and passed on with his right hand (7th). He is said to have brought the fingertips of his left hand together with the thumb, as if he were holding a raw egg. The fingertips of the middle finger and ring finger of the right hand are said to have touched the tip of the right thumb.

The little finger and the index finger were said to have stood away from the middle and ring finger at a ninety-degree angle. This is the extra technique that Usui personally liked very much. Usui raised one hand to obtain the Reiki energy and passed the same energy received with the other hand. This is the technique used by Pranic healers also.

Note – Taken from various Internet sources

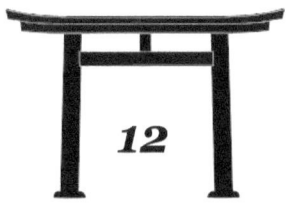

12   *Visualizations*

Gassho Meditation

Sit calmly with head upright, and eyes closed. Do Pranayama five times. Draw the symbols in your hand and do Gassho and then bring hand above the head. Visualize the hand is going to the higher planes and extracting the vibrations of light which flows into the body. Feel that you are now at one with the Universal Energy. Imagine that you are breathing through hands.

Feel the inhaling and exhaling like, extracting the positive energy and releasing the negative energy. When the hand has got enough vibration or the flow of negative energy is minimized then slowly put one hand on the heart. You can either put the right or left hand; it is according to your dominant hand position.

Now one hand is above and other is on the heart. The Universal Energy is coming in through the raised hand and releases the energy through the lower hand to the heart. It is like one hand receiving and other hand giving it. Now we can feel the energy in the heart remain there till the heart is filled with it.

You can also change the hand from heart to the problem areas wherever in the body and fill it with the vital energy. Do this as much as you like. Once you finished do pranayama 5 times and slowly open the eyes.

Symbol visualization

Sit calmly with head upright, and eyes closed. Chant OM three times. You can use any other Mantras instead of OM as per your religious upbringing. After that, watch your breath, inhaling and exhaling. Listen to the sound of breathing, in inhaling the sound is "So" and in exhaling the sound is "hum". This means I am He (the prana/soul).

If you cannot hear the sound then just watch the breathing. Imagine that through every breath you are tuning with this source. That divine energy is inhaled to stomach and exhaled from there.. After that draw CKR in your heart, then SHK and HSZSN. They are glazing in white light. The energy emits from is like the rays of sun. This fills the heart with positive energy and later on spreading to other parts of the body. Remain like that till you feel enough.

Then do Pranyama a few times and chant OM three times or the Mantra chanted before the meditation. Slowly open your eyes.

There is one more way to do Symbol meditation, which I normally teach in my class and also lots of ancient practices in Tibetan and Yogic system for Reiki Second level. Those techniques are not mentioned in the manual because it should be taught and monitored by a competent master. Get in touch with me to know more about it.

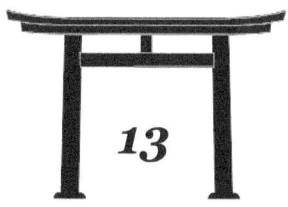

13 *Additional Materials*

Explanation Of Instruction For The Public- By Founder of Usui Reiki Ryoho, Mikao Usui

It is an old custom to teach a method to only my descendants, for keeping a wealth within a family. Especially, the modern societies we live in wish to share happiness of coexistence and co-prosperity. So I don't allow my family to keep the method to ourselves.

My Usui Reiki Ryoho is an original, there is nothing like this in the world. So I would like to release this method to the public for everyone's benefit and hope for everyone's happiness. My Reiki Ryoho is an original method based on intuitive power in the universe. By this power, the body gets healthy and enhances happiness of life and peaceful mind. Nowadays people need improvement and reconstruction inside and outside of life, so the reason for releasing my method to the public is to help people with illness of body and mind.

Q. What is Usui Reiki Ryoho?

A. Graciously I have received Meiji Emperor's last injunctions. For achieving my teachings, training and improving physically and spiritually and walking in a right path as a human being, first we have to heal our spirit. Secondly we have to keep our body healthy. If our spirit is healthy and conformed to the truth, body will get healthy naturally. Usui Reiki Ryoho's missions are to lead peaceful and happy life, heal others and improve happiness of others and ourselves.

Q. Is there any similarity to hypnotism, Kiai method, religious method or any other methods?

A. No, there is no similarity to any of those methods. This method is to help body and spirit with intuitive power, which I' ve received after long and hard training.

Q. Then, is it psychic method of treatment?

A. Yes, you could say that. But you could also say it is physical method of treatment. The reason why is Ki and light are emanated from healer's body, especially from eyes, mouth and hands. So if healer stares or breathes on or strokes with hands at the affected area such as toothache, colic pain, stomachache, neuralgia, bruises, cuts, burns and other swellings with pain will be gone. However a chronic disease is not easy, it's needed some time. But a patient will feel improvement at the first treatment. There is a fact more than a novel how to explain this phenomenon with modern medicine. If you see the fact you would understand. Even people who use sophistry can not ignore the fact.

Q. Do I have to believe in Usui Reiki Ryoho to get better result?

A. No. It's not like a psychological method of treatment or hypnosis or other kind of mental method. There is no need to have a consent or admiration. It doesn't matter if you doubt, reject or deny it. For example, it is effective to children and very ill people who are not aware of any consciousness, such as a doubt, rejection or denying. There may be one out of ten who believes in my method before a treatment. Most of them learn the benefit after first treatment then they believe in the method.

Q. Can any illness be cured by Usui Reiki Ryoho?

A. Any illness such as psychological or an organic disease can be cured by this method.

Q. Does Usui Reiki Ryoho only heal illness?

A. No. Usui Reiki Ryoho does not only heal illness. Mental illness such as agony, weakness, timidity, irresolution, nervousness and other bad habit can be corrected. Then you are able to lead happy life and heal others with mind of God or Buddha. That becomes principle object.

Q. How does Usui Reiki Ryoho work?

A. I' ve never been given this method by anybody nor studied to get psychic power to heal. I accidentally realized that I have received healing power when I felt the air in mysterious way during fasting. So I have a hard time explaining exactly even I am the founder. Scholars and men of intelligence have been studying this phenomenon but modern science can't solve it. But I believe that day will come naturally.

Q. Does Usui Reiki Ryoho use any medicine and are there any side effects?

A. Never uses medical equipment. Staring at affected area, breathing onto it, stroking with hands, laying on of hands and patting lightly with hands are the way of treatment.

Q. Do I need to have knowledge of medicine?

A. My method is beyond a modern science so you do not need knowledge of medicine. If brain disease occurs, I treat a head. If it's a stomachache, I treat a stomach. If it's an eye disease, I treat eyes. You don't have to take bitter medicine or stand for hot moxa treatment. It takes short time for a treatment with staring at affected area or breathing onto it or laying on of hands or stroking with hands. These are the reason why my method is very original.

Q. What do famous medical scientists think of this method?

A. The famous medical scientists seem very reasonable. European medical scientists have severe criticism towards medicine. To return to the subject, Dr. Nagai of Teikoku Medical University says, "we as doctors do diagnose, record and comprehend illnesses but we don't know how to treat them."

Dr. Kondo says, "it is not true that medical science made a great progress. It is the biggest fault in the modern medical science that we don't take notice of psychological affect. Dr. Kuga says, "it is a fact that psychological therapy and other kind of healing treatment done by healers without doctor's training works better than doctors, depending on type of illnesses or patient's personality or application of treatment. Also the doctors who try to repel and exclude psychological healers without doctor's training are narrow-minded."

It is obvious fact that doctors, medical scientists and pharmacists recognize the effect of my method and become a pupil.

Q. What is the government's reaction?
A. On February 6 th , 1922, at the Standing Committee on Budget of House of Representatives, a member of the Diet Dr. Matsushita asked for government's view about the fact that people who do not have doctor's training have been treating many patients with psychological or spiritual method of treatment.

Mr. Ushio, a government delegate says, "a little over 10 years ago people thought hypnosis is a work of long-nosed goblin but nowadays study has been done and it's applied to mentally ill patients. It is very difficult to solve human intellect with just science. Doctors follow the instruction how to treat patients by medical science, but it's not a medical treatment such as electric therapy or just touching with hands to all illnesses."

So my Usui Reiki Ryoho does not violate the Medical Practitioners Law or Shin-Kyu (acupuncture and moxa treatment) Management Regulation.

Q. People would think that this kind of healing power is gifted to the selected people, not by training.

A. No, that isn't true. Every existence has healing power. Plants, trees, animals, fish and insects, but especially a human as the lord of creation has remarkable power. Usui Reiki Ryoho is materialized the healing power that human has.

Q. Then, can anybody receive Denju of Usui Reiki Ryoho?

A. Of course, a man, woman, young or old, people with knowledge or without knowledge, anybody who has a common sense can receive the power accurately in a short time and can heal selves and others. I have taught to more than one thousand people but no one is failed. Everyone is able to heal illness with just Shoden. You may think it is inscrutable to get the healing power in a short time but it is reasonable. It's the feature of my method that heals difficult illnesses easily.

Q. If I can heal others, can I heal myself?
A. If you can't heal yourself, how can you heal others.

Q. How can I receive Okuden?

A. Okuden includes Hatsureiho, patting with hands method, stroking with hands method, pressing with hands method, telesthetic method and propensity method. I will teach it to people who have learned Shoden and who are good students, good conduct and enthusiasts.

Q. Is there higher level more than Okuden?
A. Yes, there is a level called Shinpiden.

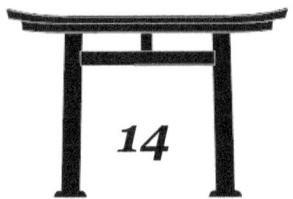

14   *Takata Handouts*

Notes from a level 1 Reiki with Takata*

(The following purports to reference a Level 1 Reiki Course held by Takata. It is attributed (rightly or wrongly) to Harue Kanemitsu, who is known to have taken both Level 1 and Level 2 with Takata. What we now call the 'Level 1' course, Takata actually referred to as the 'Introductory' course).

REIKI HEALING CLASS On August 29, 1975

It is important to somehow motivate people to also help themselves and not rely totally on the healer. This can be done by neck exercises, and I would add, by foot and hand reflexology, by prayer, and above all a fierce desire to get well. They must learn to control their feelings and thus eliminate hate and fear and anger and greed. It is a medical fact that the above feelings release deadly poisons into the human body!

It is advisable, good and practical for two or more REIKI healers to work together, to heal each other, to strengthen their mutual faith, exchange experiences, and gain confidence. Furthermore 'Where two or three are gathered together in my name, there I am in the midst of them.' Since 'REIKI' means universal power and wisdom, the above quote is applicable. Jesus was not talking of Himself, but of Universal Love and Wisdom, with which He declared Himself to be one. If you feel power only in one hand, you can hold hands with yourself and charge or warm up the other hand.

When encountering cold body areas, it is a sure indication such areas need healing (unless the man is an iceman!!) after a long enough period of laying on hands, one can then feel the vibrations and then proceed the normal way until the vibs cease, or until allotted time is up, and continue later with more treatments.

The patient does not necessarily feel tingling where the hands are laying, the tingling might be felt in an entirely different area. However the healer follows HIS or HER directions and feelings.

ALLOW LOTS OF TIME! don't become discouraged if results are not immediate. Relaxation or sleep are results of tensions vanished or diminished!

It is well to have an agreed starting and finishing time, especially when working with a number of patients.

Four of us were led into a room and asked to sit in straight backed chairs in a row. I was told to take my wrist watch off because the teacher's power would damage the watch. She then explained that it was unimportant just what we call the power nor that we know why it works, but she would show us exactly how to use it.

She then asked us to fold our hands in a prayerful way: flat palm to palm, with arms lose and relaxed, holding the hands with the thumbs about level with the third eye. We were then told to close our eyes in this position and she took up a position a few feet in front and to the left of us. We could then feel a tremendous power, almost like much static, especially in the face and the hands. While we could not see, I know she did move in front of us. Two or three times she touched our hands and perhaps she did bless or purify our fingers and hand. One time she blew strongly in our faces. Then she told us we could open our eyes. The past is over and done with. Your hands are now healing hands.

We then left the private room, and in the large living room she set up four straight backed chairs in a row, one behind the other, and we were told to sit in the chairs and begin healing another. She told us how to put our hands on the shoulders of the person in front: Put a slight pressure on the fingertips, let the palm also rest on the shoulder, and we should in our own fingertips feel vibration, and warmth in our shoulder from the contact of the person behind us. The person in front puts his or her hands in lap. After about five minutes we changed positions. All participants underwent this experience. she then went on to say that from now on we should begin to heal ourselves. Those who are overweight would lose the avoir-dupois and those who are under weight would gain up to their right weight. I believe that I experienced a healing in my right ear while sitting in the 'chair line-up.' She outlined two healing series:

1. Put both hands over eyes, with slight pressure on the eyeballs for about ten minutes, then move hands to roughly above the ears, but a little more forward, for the same 10 minutes, then move hands on back of head, just above the neck for ten minutes.

2. This series is very similar to the 'chakra-method.' You put the hands over the solar plexus, then cover the spleen, then the reproduction area, then the heart, the throat, and the forehead.

It is immaterial what you think while healing yourself or others. It does not matter how you stand or sit, just so you are comfortable. Wherever there is 'disharmony' in the other person's body you feel a vibration in the hand.

She mentioned a black lady who was a diabetic and was about to lose her eyesight, she could no longer read the newspaper, and was vastly overweight. She regained her eyesight almost immediately and within 9 months lost a lot of weight.

The instructor said she no longer uses or needs glasses, even though she wore glasses most of her life.

For a while I was sitting in front of the chair-row with the four healers in it, and I could feel the power emanating from them. I could also see the strong auras of the people, even after they left the 'healing row' their aura stayed strong. On one fellow I could see the aura not only about his head, but around his entire body.

I have a feeling that there was a connecting 'arc' of

spirit between the healers in the chair row, but could not very well ask about it.

The instructor at times is somewhat disconcerting in her answers, and I have a feeling that she does not want to give more away than she has planned.

There were about twelve in our group Paul James (ed.: name changed to protect anonymity), our host, is among them.

It was announced that tomorrow (second night) all healing pertaining everything from the neck up will be covered, including mental disturbances.

She urged that we practice healing tonight yet. (What better way to make stick what she told us. She did not want us to take notes, but rather to watch her closely. 'Distant healing' will be a graduate course, for those who have mastered what she is teaching in the basic course)

This promises to be an interesting four days! Bless the little woman.

REIKI HEALING CLASS - Second Night

Tonight's subject was everything pertaining to the head, from the shoulders up.

We again had our 10 to 15 minute private charging period. This time we were told to place our hands immediately in the praying position mentioned last night: hands flat together, arms free, especially at the body, at about the height of the 'third eye.' I felt my hands getting warmer from the wrist up, almost as if they were being filled with heat. When the heat reached my fingertips I had a tingling sensation.

- Healing the EYES: anything to do with the eyes, including glaucoma, cataracts, sties. Place a napkin (paper) over the eyes, and put fingers over the eyes, then move to the side of the head, and then back of the head. She had success in all eye diseases, some take months, others only a few treatments. It is always advisable to treat daily, for 15 to 20 minutes.
- Healing of the nose: place napkin over the nose, but do

not obstruct the nostrils, place hands over nose, then over cheekbones, and finally over forehead, and top of head.

- Healing of asthma: Place hands at root of throat, were it joins shoulders, then on underside of jaws and on cheeks, then nose as noted above. Also treat ovaries if female, or prostate if male, also solar plexus.
- Healing of ears: Place hands over ears, put finger in ear, then put patient on side and place hand behind the ear, then turn around and do same behind other ear, also treat solar plexus and throat, for ear trouble may start with wrong nutrition. Clean out ears, after treatment. Wash eyes after treatment, but don't rub them.
- Healing voice box and build up voice: Place hand (and finger) in indentation where throat joins shoulder, then treat throat all around.
- Healing migraine headaches: They are frequently caused by wrong nutrition, and thus the stomach and kidneys require treatment (see tomorrow's lecture). Then treat as if for asthma and hay-fever, also top of head, back and sides and throat.
- It was also pointed out that the feet should be treated, naturally with the shoes off.
- Loss of hair, even bald-headedness, can be treated, and it is important that proper diet be observed. Lemon juice, seeds, etc. She did not say too much about diets, but indicated the importance of it.
- Healing of teeth: Place hand over upper and lower jaws, move to cover all teeth.
- Healing of gum troubles: same way. Do not be concerned if teeth become loose, for this is part of the cleansing and healing process. The gums will tighten up again as they heal.
- Healing of the tongue and inside mouth: same way.
- Healing of goiter: (there is a visible, outer, and also and inner goiter. Trouble is caused by wrong digestion, and solar plexus and kidney should be treated first, then place hands at root of the neck, where goiter would be, then treat eyes

as outlined on page #1. Goiter will cause bulging eyes. Also treat heart, because Goiter is also a circulation problem.

- Healing of warts and Polyps: same way, by placing hands over warts and over nose (if polyps) in due time they will simply fall off, fall out including their roots. Polyps are usually cut off or burned off, but the root remains and thus they grow back in.

Today our instructor did mention that healing takes place through the power of God, and our 'REIKI-Hands' are simply channels through which the power flows.

She squeezed out all 'blackheads' on the back of our 'model' and indicated that they are signs of a too rich diet, especially too much sugar and fat.

Today, also, after our 'private session, we were sitting in the 'four chair healing parade,' as outlined yesterday. In both, the private session and the healing chairs we alternated man and women. She said we would never lose our healing power, except if we were to try and teach REIKI to another.....

She said our sensitivity would improve as we practice what we learn. When we experience the tingling sensation we encounter an area to be healed. When it stops, it is time to move our hands again. "Heal yourselves! Heal yourselves! she said several times, you come first before others.

It was brought out that there is nothing wrong with charging people for a service received, especially so since the healer invested time and money to become efficient in the work. Also the healer may have to pay for services, which he or she would normally do him- or herself if time was not taken up with healing, not to speak of cost of table, a room set aside for it. There may be other 'signs' of healing action such as diarrhea, weakness and feeling upset.

Meditation and prayer before beginning treatments is always a good way of 'focusing' the power.

It is well to check and calm the fear the patient may have. The healer may find that he or she has ups and downs in healing power, but by keeping on doing the work, this will eventually level out and up.

Sometimes one's own family simply refuses to believe that one of their own is a gifted healer, but then it has been discovered before that 'A prophet may not be welcome in his own country.' After all doctors don't treat their families either.

Heavy perspiration can also be an indication of healing taking place.

In healing, others have also had the sensation that there is no body where the healers hand is resting.

A good phrase for our type of work is SPIRITUAL THERAPY. That not only covers the laying on of hands, but spiritual counseling, even prayers and is 'non-committing.'

When both hands are placed together in this fashion a greater concentration of power is achieved.

In treating the back, place hands as indicated as keep them moving , down, down, down, on both sides, then treat the spine last, top to bottom.

A sort of X-ray healing can be achieved by placing right hand in front over disharmonious spot and the left hand in back. (if you can reach it) This is where two healers can do things one can't!

Added notes pertaining to second night (given on the third night):

- Migraine headaches: Treat feet also.
- Baby Drools: Treat head, teeth and also feet.
- Eye disease: As noted, but also treat ovaries or prostate.
- Nose Bleeding: If artery is out, pack of ice in nape of neck, pinch nose. May take 2 to 3 hours to stop.
- Lesions on Tongue, Swollen tongue: Treat head and throat, but also feet.

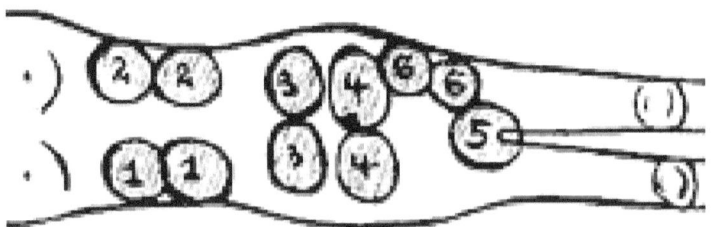

Reiki Healing Class - Third Night

The one, two, three, and four treatment: It is an almost universal treatment, and since the hands cover a rather large area, one need not be concerned about exact locations. The instructor said the Solar Plexus can be compared to the main-motor of the body, it affects all other operations, therefore keep it in A-one operating order!

- Bad breath is an indication of poor digestion (or bad teeth!)
- (6) is location if constipated.
- One can treat people, plants, animals and fish with REIKI.
- Vitalize your food (bless it, see it as God-substance, thus every meal is partaking in God-substance or is a Holy and Wholesome supper- Unity)
- Pneumonia, Tuberculosis, Cancer (anywhere), Gallbladder - always apply the 1 to 4 treatment.

Treat light cases first in order to gain confidence and to build up the healing - channel's own faith in Reiki. Never give up! R E I K I = Universal Life Energy, God-Power, Creative Intelligence.

Food: Grapefruit juice, raw beets, grated raw celery, soy-milk.

(5) indicates healing location for colons and gall bladder. Raw red beets are excellent for cancer and blood purification.

Stay away at first from third stage Hemorrhage treatments, but go ahead with second stage, however be prepared to see it get worse at first, add'l flow is indication that cleaning is taking place.

- Pneumonia: Place arms of patient behind and under head. Then with patient laying face up, reach with both hands under patient and treat one side of lungs, then stand on other side and treat that same way.

Caution : Do not uncover patient, only enough to lay on hands. If patient perspires, wash gently, always rub UP towards heart, face and throat rub down. Give liquid food. Treatment lasts as much as two hours.

- Hiccups: Put arms behind head and treat diaphragm (3&4) until it stops.
- Perma-Sneeze: Treat same as nose bleeding.
- Heart trouble is not a cause but the effect of trouble elsewhere! Treat 1 to 4, then treat the heart.
- High blood Pressure: Treat 1 to 4, then head, throat and heart.
- Emphysema: Treat 1 to 4
- Arteriosclerosis: Treat 1 to 4 and head treatments.
- Bed wetting: Treat 1 to 4 and bladder (5), then turn over and treat kidneys. Try to train not continuous urination but a sort of stop-go-stop-go-stop-go method.
- Kidneys: self treatment = stand up, reach back with both hands. others: turn around face down and lay on both hands.
- Stroke: lay patient flat on floor, ease all restricting clothing use 1 to 4 treatment, then head. If patient is lamed on one side: work downward to get blood down. Caution Left side head rules right side of body and reverse.
- Polio: Use the 1 to 4 treatment, then turn over on face and treat like common cold.
- Chickenpox: Use the 1 to 4 treatment plus head treatments (all).
- Burns: Simply lay on hands.
- Wrinkles: At young and healthy people it may indicate that the body needs more liquid! Age-wrinkles: Lay on hands, push wrinkles up and , or , in. They will then be anchored inside.
- Arthritis, Rheumatism, Dursitis, Sciatica: Use the 1 to 4 treatment, and massage the legs downward.

Instructor: ALWAYS HAVE FAITH IN GOD!

Conclusion: The REIKI Healing Method is a way of healing whereby man offers himself to be a channel for the flow of God-Power.

REIKI HEALING CLASS - Last Night

I was with the first group that went in for our usual private 'power-charge.' We were told to fold our hands in prayer and raise them as in other evenings, thumb about even with the third eye. This time I felt first a warmth in my wrist, which then slowly rose right up to my finger tips, as if my hands were forming a cup filled with heat or energy. When our instructor was standing in front of me, I felt as if my whole chest was open and a stream of gentle, but warm energy was flowing into my chest from her. She also walked behind us this time and sort of tugged at our heads, pulling it back. At the end we were informed that our healing power is permanent, we would never lose it, except if we were to try to teach or give it to someone else.

As we entered the meeting room, we again had our 4-chair line-up, healing one another. This evening dealt with the back from the neck down. While we learned the 1 to 4 of the front, we were shown today the counterpart for the back.

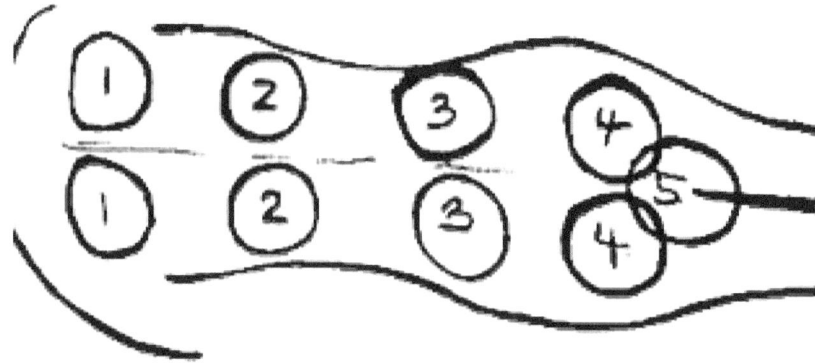

A good front and back treatment should last about 1 1/2 hours according to our instructor, and we are to stay long on the position 3 and 4 (front and back).

- For sinus, ear and nose trouble also treat the lungs above at #1 position at back.
- For whiplash treat throat, neck and back.
- For nervous breakdown: treat especially left side pos. 1 & 2 . May take three to six weeks, daily application.
- Instructor suggested that when healing is being done, that daily treatments be given.
- Important to treat spleen, which she calls the timer of the heart, Left side position of 2, 3 and 4.
- For piles and prostate gland trouble treat #5.
- For ovaries etc. treat #5
- Bleeding piles are dangerous, and cause much blood loss. Always give 1 to 4 treatment front and back and 5.
- Heart Trouble could be gas trouble, pushing against heart. Give 1 to 4 treatment front and back, then give rubbing 'back towards heart.'
- Varicose veins - treat lower body front and back and put hands right on veins.
- Watercress is good for heart trouble.
- Skin impurities have their origin in digestion, treat stomach first, then face.
- Eggs can cause itchy skin.
- Split nails - drink water-gelatin solution.
- Raw tomato juice is all right, but not the canned kind.

Our instructor emphasized again and again the 1 to 4 treatment front and back. It is important to think and use one's head: don't just treat the effect. Distinguish between cause and effect and where possible go to the cause, and I think that is why she emphasized the 1 to 4 treatment so much: it takes most everything in.

Source James Deacon's Reiki Pages

Excerpts from the Hawayo Takata's Diary *

In my attempt to write this essay on the Art of Healing in limited words, I will try to be practical rather than technical, because what I am about to define is not associated with any material being which is visible, nor has a shape, nor name. I believe there exists One Supreme being--the Absolute Infinite--a Dynamic Force that governs the world and universe. It is an unseen spiritual power that vibrates and all other powers fade into insignificance beside it. So, therefore, it is Absolute! This power is unfathomable, immeasurable, and being a universal life force, it is incomprehensible to man. Yet, every single living being is receiving its blessings daily; awake or asleep.

Different teachers and masters call Him the Great Spirit, the Universal Life Force; Life Energy, because when applied it vitalizes the whole system; Ether Wave, because it soothes pain and puts you into deep slumber, as if under an anesthetic; and The Cosmic Wave, because it radiates vibrations of exultant feeling and lifts you into harmony.

I shall call it "Reiki" because I studied under that expression. Reiki is a radionic wave like radio. It could be applied locally or as in short wave. A distant treatment could be successfully given. Reiki is not electricity, nor radium or X-ray. It could penetrate thin layers of silk, linen, porcelain or lead, wood or steel, because it comes from the Great Spirit, the Infinite. It does not destroy delicate tissues or nerves. It is absolutely harmless; therefore, it is a practical and safe treatment. Because it is a universal wave, everything that has life benefits when treated--plant life, fowls, the animals, as well as human beings, infants or old, poor or rich.

It should be applied and used daily as prevention. God gave us this body, a place to dwell, and our daily bread. We were put into this world for some purpose; therefore, we should have health and happiness. It was God's plan, so he provides us with everything. He gave us hands to use them, to apply and heal, to retain physical health and mental balance, to free ourselves from ignorance, and live in an enlightened world, to live in harmony with yourself and others, to love all beings.

When these rules are applied daily, the body shall respond and all we wish and desire to attain in this world is within our reach. Health, happiness and the road to longevity, which we all seek--I call this Perfection. Being a universal force from the Great Divine Spirit, it belongs to all who seek and desire to learn the art of healing.

It knows no color, nor creed, old or young. It will find its way when the student is ready to accept. He is shown the way. Initiation is a sacred ceremony and the contact is made. Because we are associating with Divine Spirit, there is no error; nor should we doubt. It is Absolute! With the first contact or initiation, the hands radiate vibrations when applied to the ailing part. It relieves pain, stops the blood from an open wound; your hands are ready to heal acute and chronic diseases - the human beings - the plants - the fowls - the animals.

In acute cases, only a few minutes' application is necessary. In the chronic cases, the first step is to find the cause and effect. It is not necessary to undress the patient completely, but it is better to loosen all tight clothing so that the patient may relax, lying on the table face up. Most important is to find the cause of the illness.

Start treatment from the eyes, sinus, pituitary glands, ears, throat, thyroids, thymus, stomach, gall bladder, liver, pancreas, solar plexus, ileocecum, colon, sigmoid flexure, ovarian glands, bladder, then front chest and heart. Turn patient over, treat the back, lungs, sympathetic nerves, kidneys, spleen, and prostrate gland.

During the treatment, trust in your hands, Listen to vibrations or reaction. If there is pain, it registers pain in your finger tips and palm. If the patient has itch, it reacts the same; if deep and chronic, it throbs a deep pain; or if acute, the pain is a shallow tingle. As soon as the body responds to the treatment, the acute ailment disappears, but the cause remains. Dig into the cause daily and with each treatment, improvement is seen.

After the organs have been thus treated, I finish the treatment with a nerve stroke which adjusts the circulation.

Apply on the skin a few drops of sesame oil or any pure vegetable oil. I place my thumb and fore finger on the left side of the spinal column and the three fingers and palm flat on the right side of the spinal column. With a downward stroke, 10 to 15 strokes to the end of spinal cord. Only in diabetic cases are the strokes reversed; arms and legs are manipulated towards the heart. The above treatment is called the foundation and it requires an hour or more, all depending on the complications and seriousness of the case.

Going through the body in minute detail, the hands become sensitive and are able to determine the cause and to detect the slightest congestion within, whether physical or mental, acute or chronic. Being strictly drugless and a bloodless treatment, Reiki will adjust the body to normal.

In about four days to three weeks we find a great change taking place within the body, all internal organs and glands will begin to function with much vigor and rhythm. The digestive juices put out normal flow, the congested nerves slacken, the adhesions break away, the lazy colon gets organized, the fecal matter drops from the walls of the intestines, the gases eliminate. Many years of accumulated toxin finds its way out through the pores. It is a sticky perspiration.

The bowels increase, dark and strong in odor. The urine increases like dark tea, sometimes white, as if flour stirred in water. It lasts four to six days, and yet, I have had patients who reacted with only one treatment. When this is established, you are assured of a big general overhaul of the intestinal organs taking place. With such good cleansing, the body becomes active. The numbed nerves regain sense of feeling, appetite increases; sound sleep becomes natural, eyes sparkle, skin glows like silk. With new blood and good circulation, nerves and glands restored, it is possible to rejuvenate five to ten years. At this time, it is very important what you consume.

In the Reiki health treatments, we are vegetarians, and eat all kinds of fruits in season. Nature provides with plenty, but never to waste. Over-eating is a sin. Eating in moderation, with a feeling of gratitude, to recognize the Great Spirit who is the creator, who is the All Power to make things grow and blossom and bear fruit. Come to the table with pleasant thoughts. Never eat when you are worried. Milk, white sugar, and starches are to be avoided when the patient has a weak stomach. With proper food, the patient responds faster to the treatments.

The following is another excerpt from Mrs. Takata's diary, as verified by her granddaughter, Phyllis Lei Furumoto. It tells of Takata's joy in the knowledge of Reiki. (Dated on: Dec. 10 – 1935)

Meaning of "Reiki" Energy within oneself, when concentrated and applied to patient, will cure all ailments - "It is nature's greatest cure, which requires no drugs. It helps in all respects, human and animal life. In order to concentrate, one must purify one's thoughts in words, and to meditate to let true "energy" come out from within. It lies in the bottom of the stomach about 2 inches below the naval.

Sit in a comfortable position, close your eyes, concentrate on our thought and relax. Close your hands together and wait for the sign. Kindly and gently apply the hands starting from head downward. The patient who is about to receive this treatment must purify one's (their) thoughts, feel comfortable, and (have) a desire to get well. One must not forget to feel grateful. Gratitude is a great cure for the mind. In all cases, the patient could be diagnosed just by the touch of (the) hand.

Date: April 2, 1936

Father was sick from cold and tired - gave him treatments and was able to take exam on the 7th and back to Kauai on the 10th - after seeing them off - came back with Julian to Mr. Hayashi's home - they were so nice and begged me to stay with them, so from that night on, I am staying here - this must have been my real lucky day as I come to think. I have gained so much knowledge in line of treatments that I found myself taking patients naturally.

Date: May 1

      Went to cure the 2 girls of Baron Takn; 2 days and they were cured. Mrs. Harazawa at Keio Hospital every night at 7:30 p.m. - Treatment for after operation - finds it very good and fast recovery. At the home office, patients began to increase ever since I came to them; it makes me feel good and very encouraging. What was more than pleasing was that Mr. Hayashi has granted to bestow upon me the secret of Shinje Den - Kokiyu Ho and the Leiji Ho - the utmost secret in the Energy Science. No one can imagine my happiness to think that I have the honor and respect to be trusted with this gift - a gift of a life time and I promised within me to do my utmost in regard to this beautiful and wonderful teaching that I just received - I shall promise to do what is right through sincere ness and kindness and shall regard and respect the teaching and its teachers with utmost reverence and respect.

Date: March 29, 1937

      The Law of Karma, so true according the teachings, when we meet, it is true beginnings of parting- "The Legacy left Phyllis cannot be denied. The immortality of my mother lives in the hearts of those who use REIKI."

*From the book 'Reiki, a memorial to Takata Sensei', compiled by Mrs. Alice Takata Furumoto, 1982.)

Reiki Manuals

Level Two & Three

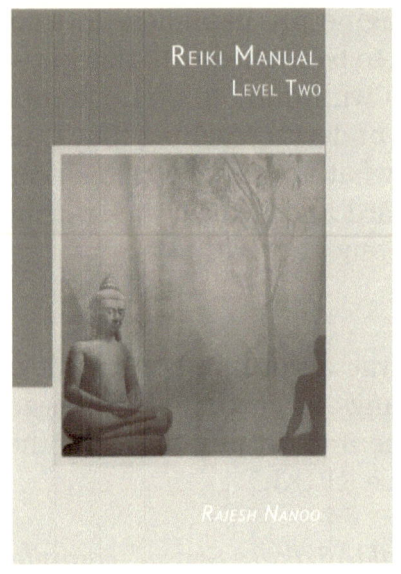
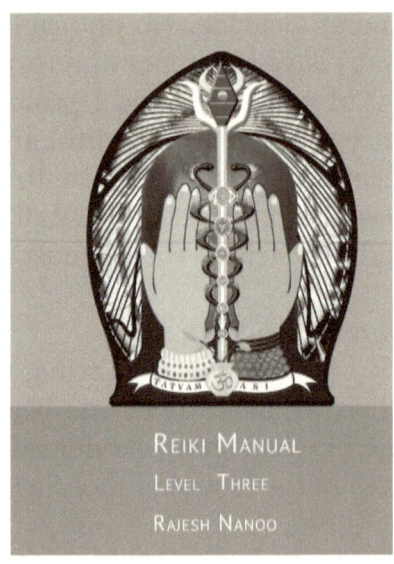

Paperbacks and EBooks are available in Createspace, Amazon, Lulu, Smashwords etc. Contact author website for more details.

www.rajeshnanoo.com

Other Books

1. The Cave Of Wisdom

The Book contains the gist of mystical teachings from Upanishads, Zen, Sufism, Kabbala, Buddhism and Taoism. Along with this, it covers the very essence of Semitic philosophy that is spread through Christianity, Islam and Judaism.

The book has many verses and stories of Upanishad exclusively translated by the author. The principal ideologies said by Upanishad Saints are shared in the book.

2. Wine Of Words

This book contains 100 short verses of progressive ideology. These thoughts aroused from Zen, Sufi, and Kabbalistic wisdom baptized in Vedantic doctrines.

3. Be......

31 mindful matters to middle path. All the good things are possible only when mind feels inspired. The whole idea of the book is to make people to be reflective and receptive towards every situations of life.

4. Reiki Sutras

Reiki the vibrational energy medicine when emitted through hands of Healer whose mind meditating on subtle love realms have the potential to relax, rejuvenate and renovate any human body and subtle bodies. The book explores the pillars and healing methodology of Reiki, which was built from the foundation laid by Saints in Indian Tantra and Lamas from Buddhism.